LIFE
WITH
FIBROMYALGIA

Fight Back With Yoga And Diet

DR. NANDA RAJANEESH

STARDOM BOOKS

STARDOM BOOKS

WORLDWIDE

www.StardomBooks.com

STARDOM BOOKS

A Division of Stardom Publishing

and infoYOGIS Technologies.

105-501 Silverside Road

Wilmington, DE 19809

FIRST EDITION MARCH 2021

Stardom Books

LIFE WITH FIBROMYALGIA/
Fight Back With Yoga and Diet

Dr. Nanda Rajaneesh

p. 146
cm. 13.5 X 21.5

Category: Health & Fitness : Diseases - Musculoskeletal

ISBN: 978-1-7369486-0-6

DEDICATION

To my family, friends and doctors who helped me cope with fibromyalgia; my husband Rajaneesh and daughter Nikita for being a pillar of strength.

My friends Bala Deshpande, Dr. Sumita Shankar and Dr. Rekha for motivating and inspiring me. Devika, Pushpalatha and Dr. Meena Kodandaram for their emotional support.

My doctors Dr. Dharmananda, Dr. Sudhir Borgonha and Dr. Raghuram for empathy and guidance.

My mother, mother in law and siblings who prayed for me.

CONTENTS

ACKNOWLEDGEMENTS

I am grateful to everyone who has helped me in writing this book.

Rajaneesh for patiently reading and editing multiple drafts.

Dr. Raghuram and Dr. Ahalya for their valuable inputs on the content of this book.

Raam Anand at Stardom Books for encouraging me to get started on this book.

Dr. Priyanka and Dr. Carunya Menon who helped me with the references.

INTRODUCTION

Fibromyalgia (pronounced as fie-bro-my-AL-gee-a), once a condition linked to other diseases or not even considered an illness, is now widely known, globally. Recent studies have also classified fibromyalgia as a disorder with reproducible pathophysiologic changes.

People with fibromyalgia suffer from widespread chronic pain, and this pain interferes with their everyday lives. The patients also experience intensified sensitivity to pain, stiffness in their muscles, fatigue, and insomnia. It takes away their enthusiasm and brings about all kinds of mood swings. In situations like these, the person has two options. Either let the pain manipulate her and push her on edge, or fight back and get her life back on track.

The illness is often seen in people who are involved in a lot of physical work. Being a surgeon, I am involved in a lot of physical work every day. As I have always wanted to be the best in my field, I was up for taking on duties any time of the day. However, once I started experiencing pain, everything turned upside down.

I looked pale and drained out of energy all the time; so much so that even my patients would come up to me and tell me that I was not the happy lady they knew anymore. My smile had vanished. My mind and body were not on the same page. While my mind wanted me to work, my body asked me to step back and take a break. I was trying to come up with reasons to excuse myself from duties, something I had never done in my entire life!

That said, I did learn an essential life-fact during this phase of my life – The human body is a well-organised biological machine that can resist every kind of environmental change. But there will be a point in life when your body cannot fight anymore; it breaks down. This is when we must take the cue and start the work on healing our body.

Many existing diseases arise out of alternation of gut organisms, bacterial infection, viral infection, some kind of autoimmune disease, or nutritional deficiencies. Getting to this level of understanding took me some time.

Chronic fatigue was one of my first symptoms, along with a persistent upper respiratory allergy. Like everyone around me, I also believed that tiredness was only a result of overworking and overstressing.

As the fatigue progressed, I felt a nagging pain in my right shoulder and upper back. A friend of mine from the orthopaedic department had warned me that the pain could be an indication of fibromyalgia. As I wasn't familiar with fibromyalgia back then, I started reading about the condition and took medications to manage my pain; my only focus was to get rid of my pain. Unfortunately, however much I tried, the pain only worsened, and I was also found to be deficient in several nutrients. By this time, along with fatigue, I was also suffering from bad brain fog and sleeplessness—I had started to lose awareness about the happenings around me. There was a huge hormonal imbalance.

I kept digging in and reading different books to find a solution, and finally, I came across a book that spoke about the connection between gluten, cheese allergy, and fibromyalgia. This was when I realised that food allergy could also be playing a massive role in my pain. It is important to follow an antioxidant diet. I have talked extensively about the importance of diet in chapter 11. It is crucial to understand the anatomical positions and pathophysiology of the musculoskeletal system. In my opinion, it is more important to know what not to do than what to do.

Once fibromyalgia hits you, you are most likely in it for life. Your muscles and tendons get worn out, and you will have to follow a strict exercise regimen to keep your body pain-free. That said, be careful with muscles where there is repetitive stress. Stretch them well. Yoga is the best practice to lengthen your spine.

Beginners should always practice dynamic yoga with proper breathing techniques. Also, find the right teacher. I had to change a lot of teachers until I found the right one. I practice yoga even today, and I must tell you, it works like a miracle.

Having said that, in fibromyalgia, along with your physical body well-being, it is also important to focus on your mental well-being. Having been independent all my life, I was suddenly dependent on people around me to function properly. My mental health was deteriorating every day. Since I was not practising, the fear of permanent loss of work also led to depression.

To everyone who is reading this book, please be patient with people suffering from chronic pain. They are already miserable, and your comments will only push them on edge. The patients will never agree to meet with a psychologist, but they need help. It is your responsibility as their family/friends to convince them that they need help.

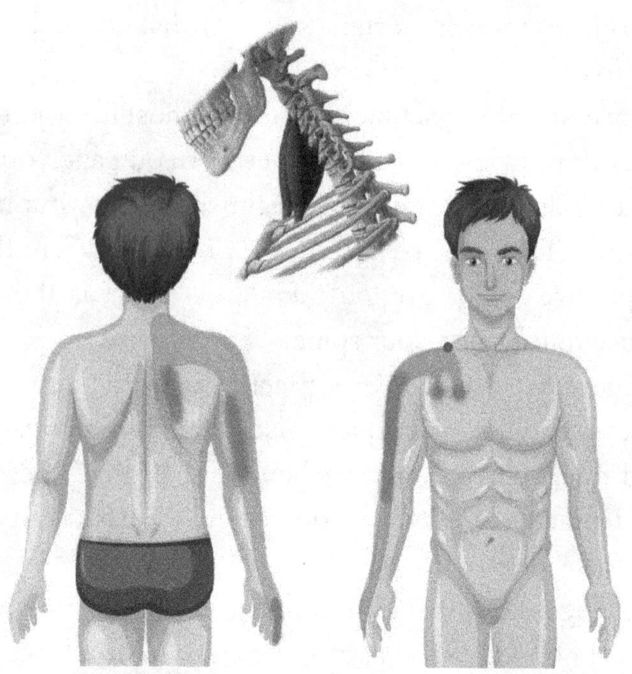

I was very hesitant initially to accept the fact that my pain was affecting my mental health; I was very sure that the pain was just physical. My family advised me to seek psychological counselling. Looking back, I am glad my family did that. Meeting with a psychologist helped me get some clarity about my condition. Although my pain continued despite the counselling, my brain fog and other psychological issues improved. It helped me gain back my self-awareness.

My friends and family were my pillars of strength. My husband and daughter were very supportive throughout the journey. I was also lucky to have the best doctors by my side; they were supportive, even though I was not a good patient. I have to mention this — one of my friends had told me never to give up on the power within me. I am very thankful for this advice, for I do not think I could have made it if I had not focused on the power within me. The patient's personal effort to heal and get better is crucial.

Summing up, I suffered a lot, but I never gave up. There were many times when I had lost all hope, but the support I received from my family and friends kept me going. I kept digging in for answers, and now, looking back, I can't help but feel proud of myself.

In fibromyalgia, our journey to look after ourselves never ends. This journey can be very tiring, but it is in our hands to make it beautiful. I have been trained in surgery from the top institutions globally, and when fibromyalgia hit me, I saw my dreams being shattered in front of my eyes. I think my dedication towards work and the willingness to be the best surgeon was one of the things that pushed me to get better.

Today, I practice breast cancer surgery and general GI surgery. I work a lot on disease prevention with an easy understanding of multiple diseases. I involve myself in teaching and practising things that do not cause much physical strain—lifestyle modification helps a lot in fighting fibromyalgia.

Suffering from fibromyalgia is like sinking in deep waters without even knowing how to swim. You need a lot of courage, support, and a lot of energy to make it to the shore. I wanted to write this book to shed light on the fact that as a doctor, even I got lost.

I recovered relatively well as I was fully aware of the anatomy of my body. I wish more people understood about fibromyalgia and its connection with gut and nutritional imbalances. If you ask me, be it any inflammatory disease, you have to consult a doctor right away. If not, there are high chances of intracellular amyloidosis. This might, in turn, lead to persistent long-term chronic disease complex!

PART A
FIBROMYALGIA: THE WHAT, WHY AND HOW

Fibromyalgia often referred to as an 'invisible disease', affects a person physically and mentally. Along with fatigue, sleep disturbances, and mood swings, patients with fibromyalgia deal with widespread muscular pain, which disrupts their daily activities. When I got to know that I was dealing with fibromyalgia, I was not very familiar with the condition. In fact, it took me a while to even realise that I was suffering from fibromyalgia.

Intensified pain, muscle tenderness, fatigue and restlessness are some of the major symptoms of this illness. These symptoms are quite common and are seen in several other diseases like hypothyroidism, anaemia, rheumatoid arthritis, Lyme disease, multiple sclerosis, and even cancer. So, it gets very difficult to diagnose fibromyalgia at the very first go. This is the reason I called it tricky earlier.

Usually, patients with fibromyalgia experience difficulties in walking, lifting and performing daily activities. Joint pain in the neck, shoulders, back, and hips are very prominent. Although fibromyalgia is not fatal, it's definitely something that will bother you throughout your life, if not treated at the right time. The pain experienced is unimaginable.

1
PAIN IN FIBROMYALGIA

"Since chronic pain frequently cannot be seen or measured, unlike acute pain, doctors, colleagues, friends or family may question or doubt your pain. In effect, it doesn't matter if anyone believes you, but it is extremely important for you to acknowledge that all pain is real."

- Pain Recovery: How to Find Balance and Reduce Suffering from Chronic Pain.

The International Association for the Study of Pain (IASP) defines pain as an unpleasant sensory and emotional experience associated with actual or potential tissue damage. The patients who suffer from chronic pain go through a lot as they cannot explain their situation to anyone. Sadly, how much ever advanced our medical field is, there is no definite cure for fibromyalgia to date.

Fibromyalgia was not considered a serious illness by anyone two decades ago. Since the pain kept shifting from one part of the body to another, many patients were accused of faking their pain.

However, in 1990, when the American College of Rheumatology first published its list of symptoms, the entire world began to learn about fibromyalgia. Currently, fibromyalgia is discussed and talked about like any other chronic illness.

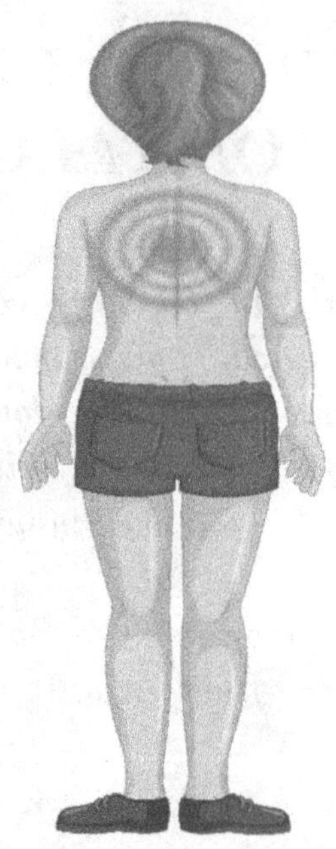

The patients with fibromyalgia often complain of a stabbing-like feeling, muscle and joint stiffness, which usually worsens when the body is idle with no movement. This is surprising because overworking and being involved in a lot of physical activity is usually seen as the root cause of fibromyalgia. But the fact that pain is experienced even while resting is what makes fibromyalgia a difficult disorder.

Here's what you need to know about pain in fibromyalgia; there are two kinds of it. Firstly, there's pain that you feel when you overwork yourself—when there's extra pressure on your nerves, the joints ache.

The second type of pain is felt when you are at rest—this is what we refer to as 'pain at rest'. I used to experience severe pain in my legs and back/spine even while I slept, and this is why cutting down on my daily work did not help me much.

Additionally, fibromyalgia is often confused with rheumatoid arthritis, because in some patients, there's swelling along with joint stiffness. This is a common misconception. Even doctors misdiagnose it sometimes. *[The importance of diagnosis in fibromyalgia is discussed in detail in chapter 12.]*

There are certain 'tender points' in our body [a muscle or a muscle-tendon junction] that ache when there's excessive pressure on them. Below mentioned are the tender points in the body –

- Neck
- Chest
- Shoulders
- Elbows
- Hips, and
- Knees

Usually, in cases other than fibromyalgia, the tender points ache for a while, and the pain is gone with a few medications; sometimes, the pain goes away by itself. However, in fibromyalgia, these places continue to hurt, no matter how many medications you take. The patients complain of experiencing shooting pains in their joints. Sometimes their pain is so intense that many patients slide into depression, not being able to withstand the pain.

So, the question here is, why do fibromyalgia patients hurt in places where there is no trace of an injury? How are all the lab reports normal? Why does the pain worsen over time? Here's an explanation. Pain amplification in fibromyalgia could be due to the sustained release of certain chemicals by the neurotransmitters like Glutamate, GABA, serotonin and dopamine.

It was towards the end of 2008 that my body started showing signs of chronic inflammation. I would be tired sooner, and I found it very difficult to even push through the day. Back then, I did not give it much thought. Being a surgeon calls for a lot of dedication; one should always be ready to take on extra work in times of need. Since over-stress could also cause all these symptoms, I got on with my life without thinking too much about it.

Towards mid-2009, September to be specific, I started experiencing shooting pain in my right shoulder and neck. But again, I neglected it; many surgeons experience such pains because of their busy schedules.

However, the pain did bother me to some extent because I had never experienced such pain in my entire life. Additionally, the pain had continued for months, and things did not look good. I used to experience severe pain in my neck and mid-back areas. But, if someone asked me to point to the area of pain, I couldn't. The situation was very new to me as well. However, I got on with my life despite the pain, and another year just passed-by.

By the end of 2010, I noticed that the pain had spread to other areas. My situation had worsened, and things got really serious in 2011 when I fainted at my workplace, while I was attending a patient.

I had to get up from my chair, but I did not have the energy in my legs. When I forced myself up the chair, I felt dizzy and fainted. The hospital staff immediately rushed me to my cabin, checked my pulse, and comforted me.

What surprised everyone and me as well, to be frank, was that I was back at work within no time. The pain just came to me, and I was all fine the very next moment!

That particular day is when it hit me that something was seriously wrong with my body and that I had to seek help immediately. I began my research. I started asking around and read a lot of books on chronic pain. Books were my main source of help around that time.

Meanwhile, one of my senior colleagues pointed out that tuberculosis also had similar symptoms and advised me to get a check-up done. It so happened that as a kid, I had spent a lot of time with my grandmother, who had suffered from tuberculosis.

So, that could have been a possibility. However, the test results revealed that it wasn't tuberculosis. Although this was a relief to me, I was worried again because the root cause of my pain was still unknown. For context, there have been a lot of studies conducted to identify the clinical effects of the BCG vaccine [vaccine that protects against tuberculosis] on the pain management in fibromyalgia. In fact, sources reveal that the U.S Food and Drug Administration [FDA] recently indicated its approval for a human clinical trial of the bacillus Calmette-Guerin (BCG) vaccine to treat fibromyalgia.

I consulted doctors all over India and abroad to understand what was happening to me. I started reading and learning about inflammation theory. I never thought my condition would worsen so much as I have always been a healthy person. I have never had any systemic problem in my entire life. I discussed my situation with another doctor friend, and he suggested I take medications.

Not being able to withstand the pain, I started taking the prescribed medicines. Although the pain reduced, the medications had their side effects; I felt drowsy and discomfort throughout my body.

I underwent all sorts of physical examinations. To my surprise, there was nothing abnormal with my body. This is one of the reasons why fibromyalgia is called an 'invisible disorder'. Everything looks fine on the outside with this illness.

After undergoing all these tests, the most common response/suggestion I got was that I was overworking myself and that stressing too much was the root cause of my sufferings. As a surgeon, I'm involved in a lot of manual work. Conducting surgeries all day long puts high amount of pressure on my hands and neck. The work also involves a lot of writing, which puts a lot of stress on my wrist.

Well, this repetitive stress could have been a reason. But normal pain usually does not last so long, even if it is caused by too much physical work.

A note to the readers: Any pain, if it is persistent and troubles you for a long time, please don't neglect it. If there is prolonged pain, it is indicating towards an underlying condition.

I was convinced there was something wrong with my body, and I had to know what it was precisely before I took the next step.

Repetitive Stress Can Cause Chronic Pain

As I mentioned before, muscles tire out very soon in case of fibromyalgia. I used to conduct multiple surgeries every day, which explains all the repetitive stress I was putting my body through.

Physiotherapy is usually the go-to treatment for this. It can help decrease the tension in the muscle and provide pain-relieving strategies. I underwent physiotherapy, and I must say, it played a vital role in helping me withstand the pain. *[I have discussed physiotherapy and other therapies that were administered in chapter 10]*

As I mentioned earlier, many researchers believe that fibromyalgia amplifies painful sensations by affecting the way brain processes pain signals. The blockage of nerve signals and nutrition supply to the cells in chronic disease leads to various diseases depending upon the damage. The root cause of all chronic diseases is subclinical chronic inflammation.

Inflammation due to autoimmune diseases or chronic infections can cause decreased connectivity between brain areas that process pain and sensorimotor signal. A 2014 study conducted in Sweden on brain connectivity had revealed fibromyalgia to be associated with decreased connectivity between pain and sensorimotor brain areas.

Another similar study conducted by Karolinska Institute, Sweden, and Massachusetts General Hospital, United States, showed that glial cells, the central nervous system's immune cells, are activated in patients with fibromyalgia. A group of researchers also believe that repeated nerve stimulation causes changes in the brains of people suffering from fibromyalgia. There appears to be an increase in certain chemicals in the brain, which results in the body overreacting to pain signals.

Since this is all internal, patients suffering from fibromyalgia are often misunderstood. This miscommunication often makes the patient feel left-out, further leading to depression in many cases *[Psychological issues are discussed in detail in chapter 3]*.

Nutrition Deficiency and Fibromyalgia:

I often flew to Delhi to attend meetings. On one such trip, I met the CEO of Onquest Diagnostics, who is also a pathologist. On discussing my situation with him, he suggested that I get a nutrition evaluation done as I complained about fatigue and tiredness.

I got the test done, and the results were quite shocking. I was deficient in vitamin D. My haemoglobin level was 6.5 g/dL *[It should be between 12.1 and 15.1 g/dL]*. My family and I were so startled that we were considering blood transfusion as an option!

Vitamin D is important for skeletal and non-skeletal health. Worldwide, vitamin D is predominantly obtained through exposure to sunlight. Latitude, cultural dress habits, sun avoidance, and sunscreen protection can all limit vitamin D production. Many patients and physicians believe that adequate vitamin D intake can be obtained via diet alone.

This assumption is erroneous. With the exception of fatty fish, the vitamin D content of most foods, including fortified dairy products, is relatively low to non-existent. Therefore, vitamin D deficiency has to be supplemented appropriately throughout our lives. Vitamin D deficiency affects intestinal health, alters regular flora and decreases immunity.

Clinical Risk Factors for Vitamin D Deficiency

- Decreased intake
  - Inadequate oral intake
  - Malnutrition (poor oral intake)
  - Limited sun exposure
- Gastrointestinal
  - Malabsorption (eg, short bowel syndrome, pancreatitis, inflammatory bowel disease, amyloidosis, celiac sprue, and malabsorptive bariatric surgery procedures)
- Hepatic
  - Some antiepileptic medications (increased 24-hydroxylase activity)
  - Severe liver disease or failure (decreased 25-hydroxylase activity)
- Renal
  - Aging (decreased 1-α hydroxylase activity)
  - Renal insufficiency, glomerular filtration rate <60% (decreased 1-α hydroxylase activity)
  - Nephrotic syndrome (decreased levels of vitamin D–binding protein)

Ref.[5]

Over the years, it has been found that patients with chronic pain disorder might also have issues with their digestive health. Fibromyalgia has been seen to be related to poor gut health. Scientists have evidence to support the correlation between chronic pains and alterations in the gut microbiome. *[Gut health has been discussed in detail in chapter 5.]*

Coming back to my story, after spending years and being unsuccessful in figuring out what was happening to me, I had started sliding into depression. Firstly, I had lost all hopes of my condition being cured, and secondly, no one, including me, could figure out what was wrong with me.

Looking at my condition, my husband asked me if I wanted to get away for some time. I did want a break from all of this. So, sometime in December 2011, my husband, daughter, and I took a trip to Goa. While my family enjoyed the trip, I was busy reading up about pain.

On December 17, I read a book on autism, where the author had talked about body pain and a condition called fibromyalgia that causes pain in different points of the body. It was at this point I figured out what exactly I was going through. Although a friend had warned me about fibromyalgia earlier, I had a clear idea of what I was going through at this point.

I had read about fibromyalgia superficially back in my undergraduate days. As I was studying to be an Oncosurgeon, I did not read much about this illness in my post-graduation. Also, a decade ago, fibromyalgia was treated mostly by psychiatrists. There was no mainstream attention paid to it. In fact, fibromyalgia was never studied separately; it was always studied with other virus infections. So, when I discovered that I had fibromyalgia, I did not know much about it.

That said, pain specialists all over the world were quite familiar with fibromyalgia. I can say this because when I consulted one of the top rheumatologists and pain specialists in Bengaluru, I was told that he was seeing more people with fibromyalgia than arthritis, and this was 10 years ago.

In conclusion, if you are dealing with chronic pain and feel fatigued most of the time, it could be related to gut health, or it could also be simple food allergies. However, if you have widespread chronic pain with severe fatigue, insomnia, and brain fog, these might be pointing towards fibromyalgia.

2
PAIN MANAGEMENT

"Pain is inevitable. Suffering is optional. Say you're running and you think, 'Man, this hurts, I can't take it anymore. The 'hurt' part is an unavoidable reality, but whether or not you can stand anymore is up to the runner himself."
— Haruki Murakami

Pain management refers to the process of easing the sufferings caused by intensified pain, which helps those with chronic pain deal with their illness and improve their quality of life.

Pain-relieving medicines, physical/psychological therapies are the different ways of managing pain. The first step in pain management is understanding the root cause of pain. Now, in the case of fibromyalgia, diagnosing is difficult. What we can do is target the basics of pain occurrence.

Why does pain occur? What cells are involved in this mechanism? Where is the highest concentration of pain receptors? and more.

For context, pain receptors, are a group of sensory neurons with specialised nerve endings that are widely distributed in the skin. When these nerve endings respond to a stimulus, pain is felt in specific areas of the brain. The degree of stimulation and the number of receptors activated define the intensity of pain.

Endorphins are basically the chemicals that our body produces to help us relieve stress and pain. Various studies have shown fibromyalgia to be associated with low endorphin levels. Thus, raising the levels of endorphins might help in managing the pain. Exercising and various massage therapies also help increase endorphin levels.

Reducing inflammation could also be one of the best ways of managing pain. Although fibromyalgia is not considered an inflammatory condition, there's evidence pointing towards inflammation playing a major role in fibromyalgia pain.

Honestly, my way of managing pain was quite strange. In the beginning, I was reluctant to take pain killers and muscle relaxants; I was worried about the side effects. However, the pain became severe as days passed, and I had no option but to resort to these medications. I was dependent on pain killers and muscle relaxants to manage my pain for a long time. As I had feared, the medicines did cause a lot of side effects — giddiness and nausea. Additionally, since I was allergic to Dicloran medication, I had no choice but to depend on Ultracet and other muscle relaxants. As a doctor, I could not help but always worry about the side effects these medicines had on my body.

When my fibromyalgia diagnosis was confirmed, I was told that Pregabalin was the drug of choice. Although Pregabalin caused a lot of giddiness in the morning, it did help me sleep well. I take this tablet even today at times and believe me, it really helps.

Pregabalin, is a widely known anticonvulsant and anxiolytic medication which is useful in treating fibromyalgia, epilepsy, neuropathic pain, fatigue, generalized anxiety disorder and many other conditions.

It was one of the first FDA approved drug to be used in the management of fibromyalgia syndrome. It has been concluded that Pregabalin can also improve global function and sleep quality in patients who have fibromyalgia.

Structure:

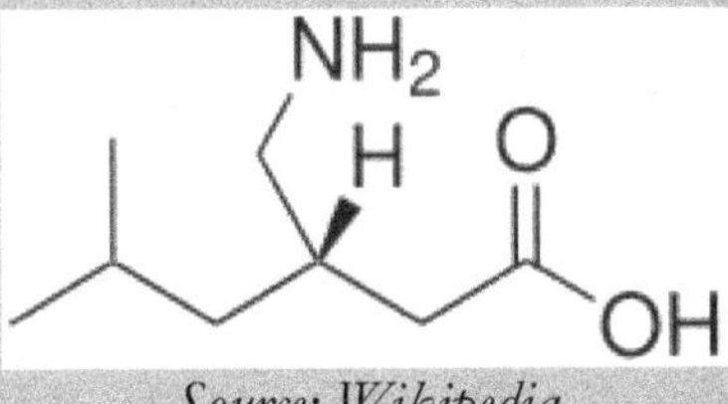

Source: Wikipedia

Chemical formula: C8H17NO2
Molar Mass: 159.229 g·mol−1

It is best if Pregabalin is administered on an empty stomach, with a Tmax (time to peak levels) of generally less than or equal to 1 hour.[1][2]

References:

1. Calandre, E. P.; Rico-Villademoros, F.; Slim, M. (2016). "Alpha2delta ligands, gabapentin, pregabalin and mirogabalin: a review of their clinical pharmacology and therapeutic use". Expert Review of Neurotherapeutics. 16 (11): 1263-1277. doi:10.1080/14737175.2016.1202764. PMID 27345098. S2CID 33200190.
2. "LYRICA – pregabalin capsule". DailyMed. U.S. National Library of Medicine. September 2010. Retrieved May 6, 2013

Known Pain Medications and Muscle Relaxants for Fibromyalgia

- Pain medications - *Lyrica*, *Cymbalta* and *Savella* are said to reduce pain and improve function in some people with fibromyalgia. They are also FDA-approved.
- Muscle relaxants - *Zanaflex* and *Flexeril.* Although there's no exact proof, these relaxants are said to reduce fatigue and pain and help the patient sleep more soundly.

Apart from using medications for pain management, I also resorted to many other forms of techniques. I took a lot of time to analyse and accept each method. I would read a lot on how each therapy helps — I tried acupuncture therapy, chiropractic care, Ayurvedic treatment, panchakarma, physiotherapy, myofascial therapy, and many more. All these techniques helped me; however, physiotherapy and myofascial release therapy were the most helpful practices.

Listed below are some of the pain management techniques a fibromyalgia patient can resort to:

- Myofascial Release
- Medications
- Trigger Point Injection
- Biofeedback
- Acupuncture
- Massage Therapy
- Treatment of Underlying Contributing Pain Generators
- Physical Therapy
- Pain Psychology

There are several studies that support the above-mentioned therapies. For instance, a study conducted in 2011 had concluded that Myofascial Release could help with the pain symptoms, physical function, and clinical severity for fibromyalgia.

I was determined to try out all the pain-relieving techniques as the pain was making me miserable. I was hoping that something on the way could help me with my pain. This is when I learned about chiropractors and their way of treating joint sprains and knots.

Chiropractic care is known to be useful for pain management in fibromyalgia for a very long time now. It effectively reduces musculoskeletal pain. Additionally, I was also of the opinion that my entire problem was purely mechanical, and that proper chiropractic treatment could actually straighten the imbalance, relieving me of this excruciating pain.

Massage therapy helped me to an extent. A good massage produces natural endorphins, thereby reducing the pain. Physical therapy is also a go-to method of pain management; it releases the stiffness in joints and muscles. Acupuncture also facilitates a good energy flow in the body.

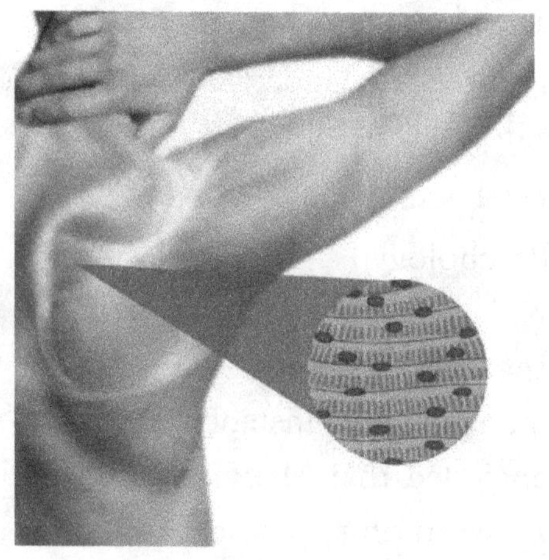

Sleep Is Essential!

Sleep is very, very important to manage pain. A recent study has confirmed that lack of sleep increases tiredness and pain. The more number of hours you sleep, lesser the intensity of the pain. Why? Well, it is said that most growth hormones are produced in our sleep. Several studies have confirmed that patients with low growth hormone levels feel fatigued, suffer from weak muscles, and have impaired cognition.

Exercise for Pain Management

An exercise program is crucial in the treatment of fibromyalgia and should include stretching, strengthening, and aerobic exercise. Although the patients might initially find it difficult because of the pre-existing body pain, one has to fight it and make it a point to get some daily workout. Numerous scientific studies have shown that exercise for fibromyalgia, especially aerobic exercise, can improve pain, physical function, and a sense of well-being.

Starting slow and sticking with the exercise program is very important. Low-impact aerobics activities such as swimming, water aerobics, walking, and biking are activities that patients with fibromyalgia find helpful. Many patients find it helpful to exercise in the morning. Some patients find yoga helpful for strengthening and stretching. A 2018 study concluded that daily-exercises help reduce pain, fatigue, number of tender points, depression, and anxiety among patients with fibromyalgia and an increased functional capacity and quality of life.

Education Is Necessary

It is necessary that there is adequate information for patients dealing with fibromyalgia. This is the sole purpose of this book. Patients should be educated about various treatment approaches, good sleep hygiene, and the importance of treating conditions that may contribute to their symptoms.

3
PSYCHOLOGICAL ISSUES

"It's all in your head" is a phrase that is commonly heard among patients with fibromyalgia. This illness has always been referred to as something to do with the mind. Peculiar thing about fibromyalgia is, since there's no one particular diagnosis, the patient ends up going through a series of screenings. And, the fact that at the end of each diagnosis, she fails to identify the exact cause of the suffering takes a toll on her mental health.

A 2018 study that explored the characteristics of psychiatric morbidity in fibromyalgia patients had concluded that chronic pain patients, irrespective of suffering from fibromyalgia were most likely to suffer from a psychiatric disorder.

Although fibromyalgia majorly refers to the physical muscular pain, the psychological aspect is very real; dealing with fibromyalgia is nothing but a rollercoaster ride of emotions. Many of my colleagues and friends suggested I visit a psychiatrist back in 2013. But I would flatly refuse saying my problems were only physical and had nothing to do with my mental health.

However, I did realise that something was wrong with my mental health. I could no longer focus on my work, my brain fog was getting worse, and I ended up getting into arguments with everyone, including my husband and daughter. Amidst all this, I even had to get a surgery near my eyeball due to an injury on my face. I was put on steroids to help me deal with the pain.

Steroids are known to reduce pain and inflammation. Although my physical pain had come down, the side effects of steroids added to my psychological issues. I started showing signs of possessiveness and hid everything dear to me, fearing it would be taken away from me.

Now that I think about it, this behaviour was mostly a reaction towards my deteriorating health. As I told you earlier, I have always been a healthy person. I could not digest the fact that my health condition was deteriorating every day. The situation was so bad that at one point, I even gave up researching and reading up about my condition. I used to sit, staring at the roof all the time. My husband would often ask me what was bothering me, but I had no answer!

Days passed, my physical situation worsened, and so did my mental health. I was on the verge of depression. Things got worse when I broke down one day in front of my parents worrying about my family's safety. I finally agreed to meet with a psychologist, and honestly, these sessions cheered me up.

I was administered Fluoxetine every day for nearly six months, along with regular counselling. My psychologist also suggested I start attending at least one patient a day. That made a lot of sense because being someone who has always dreamt of excelling in the medical field, going back to practising could distract my mind and help me regain my mental health. After about 15 sessions, my psychologist convinced me to visit a psychiatrist.

The psychiatrist listened to me for a couple of sessions, and I was very much relieved after talking to him; speaking to such a senior and experienced doctor made me feel good. After a couple of sessions, he prescribed a few basic medications, and I agreed to take it. He also counselled my husband and daughter.

The medications and sessions helped, and I was fit and fine after a couple of days. I resumed my research and got on with reading. I also resumed work eventually; it had been almost nine months since I had stopped practising.

Physiology of Stress

In pursuit of relief, we all seek various approaches and ways to deal with our external and internal pain. As mentioned in other chapters, I experienced excessive fatigue, which led to stress. Being a surgeon, I would always be a ball of energy, on my feet all day, dealing with various patients and surgeries. Additionally, I would attend many gatherings and talks post my hospital duties.

However, once fibromyalgia set in, in 2011, there were many days when I just wanted to stay at home.

This deviation in my behaviour, my dedication to work disturbed me, leading to various thoughts questioning my abilities. Thus, it is very important to understand the role of stress, especially the psychological stress that a fibromyalgia patient goes through.

Based on specific hypotheses on abnormalities of various endocrine axes and certain neurotransmitters, a possible neuroendocrine origin of fibromyalgia has also been extensively investigated. Although these systems are clearly interconnected, the potential role of the hypothalamic-pituitary-adrenal (HPA) axis lays the foundation for fibromyalgia.

HPA axis is the principal stress-response system in our body. Acute stress causes the hypothalamus to release corticotrophin-releasing hormone (CRH), which in turn releases an adrenocorticotrophic hormone (ACTH) from the anterior pituitary, leading to the secretion of cortisol, a stress hormone from the adrenals. Available medical evidence favours the diminished function of the HPA axis in fibromyalgia. Nevertheless, similar changes in most other hormones and neurotransmitters would favour a role for stress in fibromyalgia.

Brain Fog and Fibromyalgia

Fibromyalgia patients are not capable of storing and retaining information. This is termed as 'fibro-fog' or 'brain fog'.

A plausible reason for such diminished cognitive distress in fibromyalgia is derived from blunted HPA reactivity, which leads to inappropriate cortisol response to stress or activities of daily living. Due to lower activity in sympathetic and parasympathetic branches (such as higher heart rate and lower heart rate variability, blood pressure, etc.), fibromyalgia patients also displayed aberrant autonomic regulation along with reduced reactivity to physical and psychological stressors. Such an aberrant response leads to a reduced ability to face and cope successfully with environmental and daily life demands.

Moving forward, it is also seen that changes in the brain's grey matter and neurochemical abnormalities explain (at least in part) the cognitive difficulties that fibromyalgia patients complain of. Neuroimaging has found that frontal grey matter is reduced in fibromyalgia, and experimental studies have found that losses in this grey matter are detrimental to working memory processes. Indirectly, fibro-fog could also be a "downstream" consequence of changes to other brain areas that present clinically as depression, chronic pain, sleep disturbance, and a lack of concentration and attention.

Can It Be Lessened or Even Prevented?

Fibro-fog cannot be prevented per se, but a few management strategies are known to help reduce its severity. Firstly, the treatment of pain, depression, sleep disturbances, and other fibromyalgia symptoms linked to

memory loss per se, my ability to focus and learn new skills were very poor. I took up Carnatic and Sanskrit classes. My teachers were shocked to see a skilled surgeon like me lagging in her learning abilities. Nevertheless, the good news is that these deficits are not global; not all patients experience such deviation in their abilities. The severity of pain is the foremost important factor mediating these cognitive deficits. This is followed by emotional-affective issues such as anxiety, depression, and insomnia.

The Emotional Impact of Fibromyalgia

Fibromyalgia is a baggage of misery. It is linked to greater negative effects, composed of aversive emotions like sadness, fear, anger, and guilt, which are frequently associated with a worsening of symptoms, including cognitive ones.

Additionally, fibromyalgia patients display a high rate of anxiety (20%–80%) and depressive disorders (13%–63.8%). Specifically, a higher prevalence in fibromyalgia patients than in the general population was observed for generalised anxiety disorder, panic attack, obsessive-compulsive disorder, post-traumatic stress disorder, major depressive disorder, and bipolar disorders.

As a general notion, fibromyalgia patients usually feel isolated, misunderstood by relatives, friends, and society, doubling the prevalence of depression and constant and intense pain. This trauma and pain can be expressed only by the person experiencing the condition. I experienced stress as I failed to perform my duties, judging myself beyond needs, and the thought that my career could be just over. I was also constantly aware that my family members were judging me because my opinions on pain and treatment varied every week.

However, I was blessed to have a supportive husband who knew that I was a non-complaining person and that if I am complaining, the pain intensity must be quite severe. Not going off-topic, but I would very much recommend the readers to watch '*Brain on Fire*' on Netflix. I could relate to its content strongly, and it really brings out the right emotions and thoughts behind the stress and pain.

Impact of Fibromyalgia on Self-Concept

It is known that self-esteem is related to self-confidence and self-efficacy expectations. Self-efficacy is defined as the confidence in one's ability to perform or resolve a specific behaviour- this is usually low in fibromyalgia patients.

Personally, for me, reading books by the famous Indian author Deepak Chopra helped a lot in uplifting my emotional trauma. I also sought the help of yogic science, including pranayama, breathing, and asanas. Practising these have already been proven to be beneficial for various disorders.

Besides, I also adopted extensive detox therapy and Panchakarma in my routine life, which elicited a positive response in alleviating my symptoms.

During this journey, I also explored the theory of external factors influencing the internal organs, inflammation, etc. Being a medical professional, combining science and philosophy held a lot of value in understanding the bigger picture and easing my pain.

In the process, not to leave out, I invested a huge chunk of my time in reading extensively of my current stage, causes, damages, and rebound therapy for my condition. To a large extent, this with allopathic therapy, yoga, and diet helped me carve out a road to cure and prevention.

Self-Awareness Is the Key

Recognising these psychological illnesses earlier might help the patient. Firstly, tell yourself that it is okay to have all the feelings of loneliness. Self-awareness is the key. Secondly, be more positive towards life. Although continuing your hobbies might get a little difficult, try to take to them often; it helps you keep your mind off depressing things. Thirdly, let others help you. Remember, they are just trying to help you get through your situation. Consider taking a therapy; it helps get things off your chest. Additionally, know that there's someone you can go to in case you're falling apart.

SEEK HELP!

In my opinion, seeking help is very important in such conditions. My psychologist and psychiatrist saved my life. Assistance from a psychiatrist in working through these issues can work miracles. The stigma of seeking professional psychological help should be reduced. In this chapter, I have tried to address the taboo of seeking professional help. I hope that this story of how I overcame the reluctance and hesitation to seek psychological support will be of some help and can guide those struggling through such intense suffering.

That said, it is also essential to take the time to look for the right therapist, preferably someone who practices cognitive-behavioural therapy (CBT). CBT therapists focus on mindfulness. Achieving mindfulness decreases stress, and this is exactly what a fibromyalgia patient needs.

Usually, having your close ones counselling you is not a good idea, but in fibromyalgia, it is always best to have your loved ones near you. Sharing your pain with them helps lighten the emotional burden. This also helps the other person understand the position you are in.

Hope

"He who has health has hope, and he who has hope has everything."
- Thomas Carlyle

Many give up and lose hope at times, not being able to deal with the heightened pain and other unexplainable pain that they go through. As I told you earlier, I had given up. I had lost all faith in getting back to my earlier life. My advice to you is, hang in there. You will definitely make it to the shore. This is where the 'moral system' comes into play. Fibromyalgia patients who already have so much on their plates do not have to go through people telling them that 'it's just a phase' or that 'it would go away if ignored.'

On the whole, to all those dealing with this illness, remember that you are not alone. There are many out there like you. Fibromyalgia is being talked about now, and it is more common than ever. So, open up, share your story, and never, never lose hope.

4
SLEEP AND FIBROMYALGIA

It is said that a good night's sleep can do wonders. But what do you do when you don't get that good night's sleep? Well, this is simply the life of people suffering from fibromyalgia. Elika Kormeili, a licensed clinical psychologist in Los Angeles, rightly describes the pain and sleep disturbances in fibromyalgia as 'a double-edged sword.' "The more pain you have, the more difficulty you have falling asleep and staying asleep. The less sleep you get, the more of a sleep deficit you have, which makes pain worse," she says.

Sleep and fibromyalgia are interdependent. But, does heightened pain result in lack of sleep, or does lack of sleep result in heightened pain? A 2019 research published by the Journal of Neuroscience had found out that sleep deprivation had increased the sensitivity to pain by numbing the brain's painkilling response. We can thus gather that improving the patient's sleep quality may lead to significant alleviation in fibromyalgia pain. But how exactly can this be done? The key is to identify and rectify the major problems that affect an individual's quality of sleep.

Now, let me tell you a bit about my experience. I used to wake up with harrowing pain in the middle of the night and cry, not being able to withstand the pain. For me, pain definitely disrupted sleep! Painkillers and muscle relaxants helped me sleep better. I also started consuming Pregabalin regularly.

As discussed in the second chapter, Pregabalin did wonders. It reduced the pain and helped me get good sleep. I started consuming it on a regular basis and increased the dosage whenever there was severe pain. However, during my periods, the pain would not go away no matter how many tablets I consumed. I also used to suffer from insomnia whenever I experienced brain fog. I would suddenly wake up in the night, and it took hours together for me to go back to sleep.

There have been numerous studies conducted over the years on the link between fibromyalgia and sleep, and it has been found that restless leg syndrome is among the leading causes of sleeplessness in patients with fibromyalgia. Also known as Willis-Ekbom disease, the patients tend to frequently move their legs, especially at night, causing constant interruptions in sleep. A 2010 study investigated the prevalence of restless legs syndrome [RLS] in fibromyalgia. It concluded that clinicians should routinely query fibromyalgia patients regarding RLS symptoms as the right treatment of RLS can improve the sleeping habits.

Stress reduction is next on the list. We have talked about the negative impacts of stress on fibromyalgia at length in previous chapters. Destressing helps clear the mind and makes way for a full night's sleep.

The third on the list is increasing your vitamin D levels. This has been extensively discussed in the earlier chapters. Vitamin D in our bodies impact both quality and quantity of sleep. A good amount of vitamin D results in less morning tiredness, less pain and stiffness, decreased anxiety and depression, better sleep quality, and less daytime fatigue.

How Can A Patient With Fibromyalgia Achieve A Good Night's Sleep?

There are numerous ways in which a fibromyalgia patient can sleep peacefully.

1. **Exercise:**

Exercising makes way for better sleep, eases stress and restless legs, and has many other benefits. Patients should consult a physiotherapist or a yoga tutor before they start working out. Since fibromyalgia patients already have heightened pain, low-impact aerobic activity such as walking, cycling, and climbing stairs, would be best initially. The intensity of these workouts can be increased over time, depending on the individual's ability.

It is best to exercise in the morning, as working out in the morning is proven to be beneficial in getting a good night's sleep.

2. **Avoid Daytime Sleeping:**

Patients with fibromyalgia might feel the need to rest and lay down during daytime. The fatigue and tiredness will push them to take a nap; however, this might be one of the reasons for their insomnia.

Follow a sleep schedule, and in order to follow this schedule, the patients should cut down on their daytime naps. Limiting caffeinated beverages, alcohol consumption, and quitting smoking also help in following this schedule.

3. **Be Aware of Your Prescribed Medications:**

There are several proven medications that can help in improving the patient's sleep quality. One of the recent studies had also revealed that vitamin D supplements, when taken with Trazadone, an antidepressant medication, were successful in alleviating painful symptoms and improving sleep quality among people with fibromyalgia.

Before consuming these tablets, one must be aware of its side effects, as people with fibromyalgia are often sensitive to medications.

So, it is essential that the patient keeps a check on what tablets she consumes and consult the doctor before consuming any over-the-counter sleep/pain medications.

4. **Music Can Help Sleep Better:**

Listening to soothing sounds or a melodious song that the patient likes before going to bed may benefit in sleeping better.

5. **Tai Chi And Other Mind-Body Practices Might Also Enhance Sleep:**

Mind-body practices like tai chi combine meditation with slow, gentle movements and deep breathing. Practising these techniques reduces stress, and makes way for better sleep by reducing the pain.

6. **Cognitive Behavioural Therapy [CBT]:**

Cognitive Behavioural Therapy has been proven to be very efficient in treating sleep-related issues. This program helps the patient identify and replace thoughts and behaviours that cause or worsen sleep problems with habits that promote sound sleep.

It helps in controlling, if not eliminating, the negative thoughts and worries that keep the patients awake at night. In other words, it helps the patient get rid of behaviours that keep the patient from sleeping well.

7. **Practising Meditation Can Also Help Sleep Better:**

Mindful meditation helps fibromyalgia patients with sleep problems.

8. **Sleep Hygiene Is Important:**

Practising proper bedtime manners is important. Try

and limit exposure to light and noise during bedtime. Also, avoid staring at your electronic gadgets before going to sleep.

5
DOES IT START FROM THE GUT?

I was experiencing excruciating abdominal and body pain in 2011. I was also dealing with severe issues in my gut—these symptoms collectively made a case for a gut-related syndrome. I learnt about the harmful effects of gluten on the gut when I was on vacation in Goa.

Although I made significant changes in my diet, the irritation in my gastrointestinal tract was increasing, and in 2014, I finally got a colonoscopy done. Nothing unusual was seen in the diagnosis.

By 2015, I was in a very bad shape; my symptoms were more severe than ever. I got another colonoscopy done, and this time, a few ulcers were present in my distal ileum and ascending colon. Was it non-specific ulcers, Tuberculosis, or Crohn's disease? We weren't sure. My gastroenterologist suggested I take a course of TB medication for six months; that did not help.

The ulcers had increased due to the repeated colonoscopy. I was then treated for Crohn's disease with local steroids. This helped, and my condition started improving. The problems associated with my gut gradually came down, but my muscular pain did not reduce.

It was only in 2017 that my muscle pain started reducing after I learnt about the connection between food allergy and inflammation. My life became much simpler, and I could manage my pain effectively once I started a few diet modifications.

This dietary change resulted in significant relief. This led me to believe that gut theory, a causative change in gut microbiome induced by diet or pathological pattern, can definitely resolve muscular, UTI like symptoms, restlessness etc., seen in fibromyalgia.

Gut Theory: A Possible Cause of Fibromyalgia

With my recent experiments with dietary modifications, I am mostly convinced that fibromyalgia is majorly driven by gut dysfunction. After keenly observing my patients with fibromyalgia, I discovered that many of them had gut infections, dysbiosis, small intestinal bacterial overgrowth (SIBO), and leaky gut.

To further analyse this connection in the scientific literature, I reviewed several research studies connecting fibromyalgia with problems in the gut.

For example:

- 73% of patients with fibromyalgia reported GI symptoms, compared with 37% of those with osteoarthritis.
- Irritable Bowel Syndrome (IBS) is present in 30–70% of fibromyalgia patients.
- 33% of IBS patients meet the diagnostic criteria for fibromyalgia, compared to just 4% of control subjects.
- Up to 50% of patients with fibromyalgia have functional dyspepsia, which is a fancy term for "indigestion" with no known cause.

Although these correlations were quite intriguing, the research per se didn't shed much light on what actually might be causing the fibromyalgia. For me or any clinician, it is always important to understand the underlying mechanism, because addressing that root cause would enhance the effectiveness of treatment. Hence, my quest towards this goal continued, and I hit the jackpot. There were a plethora of research papers associating fibromyalgia with specific mechanisms of gut dysfunction.

Gut Theory: Cause or Effect?

One might ask "Is fibromyalgia causing these gut problems, or is it the other way around?"

The answer I found was in a study that directly addressed this question in which a group of patients with fibromyalgia, positive for SIBO were split into two groups: one group received antibiotics to treat the SIBO, the other group received a placebo.

A significant improvement of fibromyalgia symptoms was observed in the patients that achieved eradication of SIBO with antibiotics, whereas no improvement was seen in patients who took a placebo or who still tested positive for SIBO after the antibiotics. This suggests that SIBO plays a causal role in fibromyalgia for at least some patients.

Gut, The Home to Our Immune System

Inflammation is often present if there is pain, and is associated with various chronic diseases. The majority of our immune system is present in our gut (>70%) because the first wave of attack from bacteria, fungi, viruses, toxins, and even allergic food particles happens in the gut. A healthy and robust immune system is our defence against inflammation and pain. Therefore, a healthy gut is crucial to maintain optimal health.

The Gut-Joint Connection

By now, I had understood that diet does play a crucial role in maintaining the delicate balance of our microbiome. When alterations of our microbiome are compromised, there is a microbial imbalance, leading to a variety of illnesses ranging from fibromyalgia, inflammatory bowel disease and even, cancer. This is not only observed in the gut but also in parts of the body where no direct anatomical connection exists. This new area of science is beginning to identify "gut-related axes." Of particular interest is the existence of a gut-joint axis and its relation to musculoskeletal pain.

As in fibromyalgia, obesity is also a disorder of chronic low-grade inflammation resulting in increased intestinal permeability. Pro-inflammatory cytokines are known to disrupt tight junctions, impairing the intestinal barrier. The primary considerations causing inflammation are:

- Excessive absorption of bacterial cellular debris
- Poor/malabsorption of nutrient
- Intestinal permeability or leaky gut

With a leaky gut, all antigenic material (mainly food antibodies/allergies, and microbes) passing through the lining of the intestine and into circulation can get into joints, tendons, muscles, and ligaments. This hypothesis would thus reveal a strong link between fibromyalgia, inflammation, and our microbiome.

Do I Have A Leaky Gut?

Let me try and explain in simple words what a 'leaky gut' is. Anatomically, our gut is a barrier between the inside of the body and the outside world. An inner lining of intestines is a physical barrier, controlling what is absorbed and allowed to pass through. It is, therefore, crucial to maintaining the integrity of this barrier. The cells of the gut's inner lining stand side by side, forming a "tight junction" that doesn't allow anything to pass in-between except for food particles that are thoroughly digested.

When these tight junctions begin to break down, it is known as "intestinal permeability". The barrier of the gut inflames and develops holes allowing the passage of bacteria, toxins, and undigested food particles. This permeability is referred to as "leaky gut syndrome."

I strongly believe that mainstream medicine does not recognise leaky gut as a contributing factor to fibromyalgia. However, once you heal the leaky gut, the benefits are amazing.

Several conditions point to a leaky gut: Digestive issues (bloating, gas, diarrhoea, constipation, reflux), allergies or asthma, autoimmune diseases, chronic joint and muscle pain or fatigue (fibromyalgia), depression, anxiety, food allergies and intolerances etc.

Leaky Gut and Autoimmunity

In the United States, leaky gut or intestinal permeability is a critical factor in approximately 50 million patients who suffer from an autoimmune disease. With as many as 80+ different types of autoimmune diseases, the following factors are needed for autoimmunity to develop:

1) A genetic predisposition.
2) A trigger.
3) Leaky gut.

By sealing a leaky gut, you will put out the fire that feeds your inflammation, calm your immune system, and decrease your pain. Based on my personal journey with fibromyalgia, I propose the following steps to heal and manage:

1. **Glutens Gotta Go**

   In a study conducted in 2014, when 20 patients with fibromyalgia avoided gluten for between 5 and 31 months, it was seen that 15 patients got relief from widespread chronic pain, and three were able to stop using opioids altogether. Another research finding from 2017 revealed that people with signs of both fibromyalgia and gluten sensitivity responded well to a gluten-free diet.

   In 2018, scientists proposed that there could be a link between fibromyalgia and nonceliac gluten sensitivity. A 2016 paper in the Journal of Clinical Rheumatology supported the hypothesis of non-celiac gluten sensitivity and its association with fibromyalgia, spondylarthritis, and various autoimmune conditions. Gluten not only affects your musculoskeletal system and creates pain, but it also affects your nervous system.

- **Gut healing nutrients**

  Maintaining a healthy gut is the key to maintaining overall wellness. Poor gut integrity, such as the leaky gut, ulcerations, and other damages, can easily lead to food sensitivities and compromised nutrient assimilation. Amino acids, such as L-Glutamine, are known to heal the leaky intestinal gut and restore the function of the intestinal lining. Additionally, nutrients such as N-acetyl-glucosamine help to promote optimal gastrointestinal function. A gut-healing formula offers support for optimum gastrointestinal health and function including:

- Rejuvenation of intestinal mucosal health.
- Promotion of proper intestinal function.
- Healing for ulceration and inflammation

- **Powerful Probiotics**

  As I have been insisting on the fact that changes in the microbiome of the gastrointestinal tract increase the permeability of the GI tract, you must now be aware that food sensitivities are among the factors that may cause or aggravate fibromyalgia. On the other hand, I also realised that dietary deficiencies might render me more susceptible to inflammatory conditions and disorders of the immune system.

  The beneficial flora of the microbiome 50-100 CFU's probiotic with combination Bifidobacterium lactis and Lactobacillus rhamnoses will help restore the microbiome, decrease inflammation and modulate healthy immune function.

2. **Sugar**

Reducing or eliminating sugar has been the ultimate trick in resolving various lifestyle-related disorders. Consumption of foods high in sugar is linked to increased fibromyalgia pain.

3. **Carbohydrates**

There is a significant increase in the consumption of refined carbohydrates, such as cookies, slices of bread, and pastries. I often experienced an immediate increase in the intensity of fatigue and pain of fibromyalgia with the consumption of these refined carbohydrates. I would strongly recommend the consumption of simple carbohydrates such as rice or whole wheat grain.

4. **Unhealthy fats**

Vegetable oils, such as corn oil, safflower oil, and peanut oil, have an inflammatory effect, especially when used to fry food. The medical literature has linked fried foods to worsening of fibromyalgia symptoms. Other foods and ingredients that may cause symptoms for some people include, but are not limited to:

1. Red meat
2. Fruits and vegetables, such as tomatoes, white potatoes, green peppers.

3. Dairy products
4. Eggs
5. Caffeine

A Few Things to Keep in Mind

- Avoid foods, medications (e.g. antibiotics), and chemicals (e.g. BPA) that irritate the gut.
- Consider taking a probiotic and/or a prebiotic supplement.
- Treat any intestinal pathogens (such as parasites) that may be present.
- Manage your stress (with meditation, mindfulness practise, biofeedback, etc.).
- Get at least 7–8 hours of sleep each night.

PART B
VULNERABLE AND HIGH-RISK PATIENTS

Gender, age, lifestyle practices, immunity – all these play an important role in determining the vulnerable and high-risk patients of fibromyalgia. The general perception is that fibromyalgia can affect people of all age groups. Several kinds of severe physical and emotional trauma can trigger this illness. However, to date, it is mostly diagnosed in elderly people, especially women. Additionally, some studies have also revealed that genetic factors may play a significant role in causing fibromyalgia.

6
WHO IS MORE PRONE TO THIS ILLNESS?

Elderly people, those suffering from Lupus/Rheumatoid Arthritis, physical/emotional trauma, and women are seen as the primary targets of fibromyalgia. Obesity, family history and stress also play a major role in this illness.

Major Causes of Fibromyalgia:

- Repetitive injuriess
- Prolonged cough and body aches
- Emotional stress
- Viral-bacterial infections
- Autoimmune diseases
- Anxiety and depression
- Insomnia

- Hormonal imbalance
- Nervous system malfunctioning
- Obesity
- Smoking, alcohol and drug addiction
- Arthritis or other joint-related conditions
- Poor diet
- Sedentary lifestyle

Symptoms of fibromyalgia vary from person to person. Also, not all these symptoms necessarily indicate fibromyalgia. Shooting pain could also be an indication of arthritis. So, the question is when should one consult a doctor? And how can one identify if one is suffering from fibromyalgia? Additionally, since it is an 'invisible disease,' how is the illness exactly diagnosed? This chapter makes an attempt to answer all these questions.

In my experience, I have observed that a few pre-existing allergies to drugs may lead to fibromyalgia—I was allergic to drugs Dicloran, Ofloxacin, Metronidazole and Azithromycin. Usually, those suffering from recurrent respiratory infection are prescribed these antibiotics, but, if they are allergic to the administered drugs, they might end up with a gut leak syndrome.

These changes in gut organisms result in the suppression of immunity of the body, which makes the body vulnerable to diseases. So, we can say that chronic diseases may lead to fibromyalgia.

Severe leg pain, lower back pain, intensified shoulder pain and bad menstrual cramps were some of my main symptoms. These intensified towards the end of 2010, and I started experiencing heightened pain; I could feel the pain shift from one area to another.

All this continued for almost a year and a half. I was still conducting around three to five surgeries per day. Why was I overworking despite the pain? Well, I have always wanted to excel in my field as a surgeon. Having received training from reputed institutions around the world, I could not just let my pain hinder my work. Therefore, although my body was asking me to take a break, I went on with my daily duties at the hospital. I continued attending to patients and even conducted surgeries.

I turned to my colleagues and started collecting information, reading about different diagnoses and treatments based on my symptoms. Many told me that the pain was simply because of all the overwork and extra stress that I was putting my body through. Deep down, I knew that although stress was one of the causes, it could not be the main reason for this illness.

Does Gender Really Play a Role Here?

There are no specific theories to support the increased occurrence of fibromyalgia in women, but many believe that women are more prone to this illness because of their low pain threshold and their hormone structure. Many studies have also shed light on the prevalence of fibromyalgia in women who are in their child-bearing years. However, till date, there is no concrete proof to confirm the role gender-specific hormones such as oestrogen, progesterone, or testosterone play in fibromyalgia.

Neuroinflammation and Fibromyalgia

The root cause of all chronic diseases is subclinical chronic inflammation. Chronic inflammation is also the root cause of ageing. It leads to fibrosis and loss of elasticity of blood vessels, which in turn renders the tissues inefficient.

In my opinion, the mechanism by which an infection leads to fibromyalgia is very much related to inflammatory or autoimmune changes. The glandular system, nervous system and muscular system are the three main systems affected by inflammation.

Several studies over the years have revealed the presence of neuroinflammation in patients with fibromyalgia.

Additionally, the brain scans of many fibromyalgia patients indicate the pain nerves to be inflamed and irritated. The brain's pain-processing areas are found to be out of communication with one another, leading to various physical impacts on the body such as fatigue, shivering, and all the other symptoms we discussed in previous chapters.

A couple of findings have also shown the possibility of treating fibromyalgia by targeting the neuroinflammation. Again, there have been no conclusive results, and the research is in progress.

My Observation About Inflammation and Healing Process in Patients with Fibromyalgia

One might wonder about the link between inflammation and healing, and what any of these have to do with fibromyalgia in the first place. Well, here's an explanation. Blockage of nerve signals and nutrition supply to the cells in chronic disease leads to various diseases depending upon the damage. As I said earlier, the root cause of all chronic diseases is subclinical chronic inflammation.

Usually, in any excessively growing cellular area such as the antenatal injury, injury to the skin, or superficial intestinal injury, healing happens without scarring. However, in other slow-growing organs such as skin, muscles and ureter, the healing ends up leaving a scar.

Now, neuronal activity is dependent on the electrical potential in tissues. For context, our body is active due to nervous system signals and self-signals from the DNA. Furthermore, whatever be the cause of the inflammation, it mainly affects the glandular system, nervous system and muscular system.

As chronic inflammation leads to fibrosis and loss of elasticity of blood vessels, the nerves travelling in these tissues lose the capacity to carry signals.

Imagine the pathway of capillaries and nerves around the normal active cell. Capillaries give nutrition, and nerves send/receive signals. When there's inflammation, the pathway is altered, leading to changes in receiving the signals and nutrition.

It also further leads to accumulation of toxic products (oxidants), which in turn might damage the cell; the damage can be either mild or major.

Mild Damages

Mild damages could be the changes in receptors on the surface of the cell or swollen cell (hypertrophy), less active and fatigue of cell (fibromyalgia), even excessive accumulation of adipose tissue (fatty liver).

Major Damages

A major form of damage could be the death of the cell(apoptosis), islet cell death(necrosis), hypertrophy (multinodular goitre) or mutation with excessive growth (malignancy).

Now, I have a few questions based on what we have discussed so far with regard to inflammation.

- How exactly does inflammation in the body disturb the neuronal activities in the body's muscular and glandular systems?
- Does the scarring of tissues trap the nerves and blood vessels?
- Is there an entity of subclinical inflammation?
- Is inflammation the cause of all glandular diseases?

- Is chronic inflammation and healing the cause of ageing?
- Does the principle of physics that govern the existence of mass apply to human existence? Does change in density of tissues cause loss of neuronal control on the cell?

Although there are no definitive answers to these questions, they are in itself enough evidence to prove the fact that neuroinflammation exists in patients with fibromyalgia.

Obesity and Fibromyalgia:

Obesity, which is a burning issue worldwide, has long been validated as a risk factor that could lead to fibromyalgia.

Hormone Imbalance and Firbomyalgia:

Hormonal imbalance is also associated with the deficiency of nutrients/vitamins in patients with fibromyalgia. To enumerate, the major endocrine glands include the pineal gland, pituitary gland, pancreas, ovaries, testes, thyroid gland, parathyroid, gastrointestinal and adrenal gland. The endocrine system is in contrast to the exocrine system, which secretes its hormones to the outside of the body via ducts; the glandular system also contains smooth muscle around ducts and glands.

Now, inflammation can lead to spasm of these smooth muscles. Secretory activity is dependent on the autonomic nervous system and is equally important in the supply of all nutrients.

This is the main reason why hormonal imbalance is associated with deficiency of nutrients/vitamins in fibromyalgia [*Hormone imbalance and fibromyalgia has been discussed in detail in chapter 8*].

Other Causes:

One of the studies conducted in the mid-1980s had revealed the prevalence of a specific gene in fibromyalgia patients. Although there are not many studies confirming the genetic transfer of this disorder, it is something to watch out for.

Over the years, it has also been found that viral infections like the influenza virus and various upper respiratory infections may cause fibromyalgia. A 1997 study had shown many fibromyalgia patients to have a history of acute febrile and congestive respiratory episodes prior to the onset of their illness; Influenza virus infection was seen as a possible contributory factor in fibromyalgia.

A few other studies have talked about possibilities of herpes simplex virus (HSV), AIDS and hepatitis being linked to fibromyalgia.

Several researchers have also revealed that bacterial, yeast and parasite infections can cause this disease. So, answering the question of who is more prone to fibromyalgia, it is safe to say that this condition can occur in anyone from children to the elderly.

When Should One Consult a Doctor?

As discussed earlier, the symptoms of fibromyalgia can mimic those of other medical conditions, so getting it diagnosed as soon as one experiences the previously discussed symptoms is a good way to go about it.

7
IS IT MORE COMMON IN WOMEN?

Yes, fibromyalgia is more common in women. National Institute of Health (NIH) had revealed in 2015 that around 80-90 per cent of fibromyalgia diagnoses were in women.

Even today, career-oriented women are expected to wake up early and tend to the entire household in many families. Insufficient sleep often leads to fatigue, in turn resulting in heightened sensitivity to pain. A 2017 study had revealed that 49 per cent of women with fibromyalgia had a rough life, either physically or emotionally.

Below-mentioned are some of the commonly seen symptoms in women with fibromyalgia:

- Irritable bowel syndrome
- Drowsiness
- Sleep disorders

- Anxiety, depression, and other psychological issues
- Joint aches
- Frequent mood swings
- Stomach related disorders.

Fibromyalgia is more common in women who are into a lot of physical work. Back then, I was conducting multiple surgeries per day, and I also did a lot of paperwork. There was too much repetitive pressure on my neck and shoulders. Too much repetitive physical stress leads to knot formations in our body, which are felt just under the skin, causing pain. When this pain intensifies, the patient experiences physical weakness.

Several other studies confirm that women suffer from chronic fatigue and irritable bowel syndrome more often than men which supports the fact that women have a relatively weak immune system and higher pain sensitivity.

Why Exactly Are Women at A Higher Risk?

As we already know, hormones are what makes females different from males. Females produce oestrogens, and progesterone from the ovaries and various studies have revealed that the higher the oestrogen levels, the more hyperactive a subject becomes.

Excessive progesterone can make the subject more tired. This oestrogen dominance has long been discussed with respect to chronic illness and other autoimmune conditions.

This very difference in hormones is the reason for men and women reacting differently to stress. The increased hormonal activity in women under stress becomes the main reason for them being at a higher risk of fibromyalgia.

On the other hand, researchers have asserted that the endorphins are released more effectively in men, thus activating the pain-killing receptors.

Now that we know why women are more prone to this illness; let's look at the major trigger points in women with fibromyalgia.

- Neck joint
- Shoulders and arms.
- Forearm
- Side of the breastbone
- Hips and lower back
- Uterus and pelvis, while menstruating
- Knees and legs

How Common Is Fibromyalgia in Men?

Though the cases are few, a significant number of men do suffer from fibromyalgia. Since women are known to be at a higher risk, doctors end up ruling out fibromyalgia in men. So, lack of testing may have led to fewer cases in men.

Men who fly a lot can also be at a higher risk of fibromyalgia. When there is less oxygen supply to the muscles and joints in our bodies, they start to ache. In cases like these, oxygen therapy is generally advised to the patients. Studies have revealed that higher oxygen intake could improve people with fibromyalgia and chronic fatigue.

In addition, studies have suggested that cultural factors like toxic masculinity may also play a role. For example, it is generally thought that feeling pain is normal among women. However, a man is not expected to show his pain. So, men who have fibromyalgia hide their pain and refrain from consulting a doctor.

Is There Any Difference in The Way Men and Women Are Affected by Fibromyalgia?

Yes. There is. In chapter 3, we learnt about the psychological effects of fibromyalgia in women. Men with fibromyalgia also deal with a lot of psychological issues. As fibromyalgia makes them weak and moody, it affects their mental well-being, which directly affects their careers. Now, there are some families where men are the sole breadwinners. In such cases, taking care of the family becomes a difficult task.

A nationwide survey conducted by the American Journal of Men's health in 2018 had revealed that this lack of understanding among close family and friends and in the workplace might put a man with fibromyalgia in a very difficult spot.

In situations where men are supposed to be strong, not share their pain, or sit idle at home, it gets really difficult to manage a condition like fibromyalgia. The high expectations add on to their emotional grief, and this might push a man onto the edge.

Remember, diseases do not hit you, considering your gender. Although it is said that men can withstand pain, a disease like fibromyalgia will eat a person from the inside if it is not dealt with at the right time. So, irrespective of gender, a person with fibromyalgia should be provided with good care and should be treated with love and affection.

A 2017 study that evaluated the gender differences in patients with fibromyalgia had revealed that there was a higher frequency of hyperalgesia in women and that this was the only feature that makes the prevalence of fibromyalgia more common in women. It had also noted that there was no statistically significant difference found in men and women in terms of fatigue, sleep and mood disorders.

On the whole, the gender differences in fibromyalgia are still being studied. Although there are no conclusive results yet, one thing is definite - the psychological and socio-cultural factors have a huge role to play in fibromyalgia

8
IMPACT ON THE HORMONAL ACTIVITY

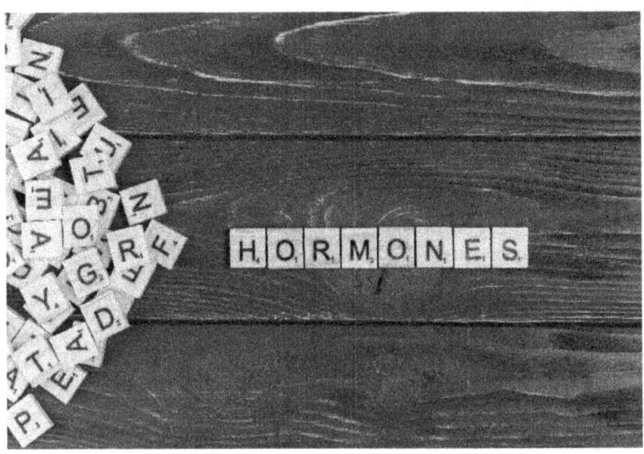

The hormonal activity has an impact on fibromyalgia. The fact that women with fibromyalgia experience heightened pain during their menstrual cycle further confirms this theory. The sex hormones not only affect the activity of pain receptors in men and women but also the pain processing pathway in the nervous system. For context, hormones are your body's chemical messengers. These powerful chemicals, produced in the endocrine glands, travel around your bloodstream, telling tissues and organs what to do. They help control many of your body's major processes, including metabolism and reproduction.

What is Hormonal Imbalance?

There are times when our body makes too much or too little of specific hormones. This hormone imbalance affects both men and women differently. Hormone imbalance is common if you suffer from endocrine disorder.

What Causes Hormone Imbalance?

Medical conditions such as type 1 and type 2 diabetes, and other thyroid disorders are associated with different hormone imbalances. While menstrual changes are the major contributors to hormone imbalance in women, hypogonadism can be the cause in men. Stress also plays a crucial role in hormonal imbalance.

Hormonal Imbalance and Fibromyalgia

Several studies over the years have confirmed the link between fibromyalgia and low serotonin, noradrenaline and dopamine levels in the brain. As these hormones play a major role in regulating our mood, appetite, sleep and behaviour, it can be deduced that hormonal imbalance aggravates the symptoms of fibromyalgia. Additionally, these hormones in the brain also play a role in processing pain signals. An imbalance in the level of hormones produced can result in heightened sensitivity.

Now, coming to the question of why women experience heightened pain during their menstrual cycle, here's an explanation based on my own experience. I have always been a healthy person. Not once in my life, until 2011, had I experienced menstrual cramps or premenstrual syndrome [PMS]. At the beginning of 2011, I started to feel a bit restless and vulnerable during my periods. Initially, I did not give it much thought. However, as days passed, my cycles started becoming irregular; they were delayed. And, when I got my periods, I suffered from terrible cramps.

Although I managed the pain by popping painkillers initially, it got worse over the months. It was so bad that I would roll on the floor in the middle of the night, screaming with pain. I could not stand or walk. Additionally, the pain was not just in my pelvis. It was throughout my lower body. Now that I think about it, the heightened pain could have been a combination of both menstrual cramps and fibromyalgia.

That said, I should tell you that I also had a retroverted uterus – meaning, my uterus was tipped backwards and was falling on the rectum and not the belly. This resulted in constipation, bloating, gas, and many other complications. In 2012, I visited my gynaecologist, and after an informed discussion, the doctor performed a hysterectomy and removed my uterus.

The common conception is that fibromyalgia worsens when the woman has her uterus or ovaries removed, but I can't entirely agree with this view. Although I still had pain in my pelvis, the surgery certainly did not contribute to anything worse. If anything, I was relieved from my uterine and menstrual pain.

Additionally, hormone imbalance resulted in irregularities in my eating, sleeping, and thinking patterns. I was also getting night sweats. Talking about night sweats, I get them even today whenever I eat cashews, almonds, lentil, flaxseeds, and cornflour. I am 49 now[at the time of writing], and if I go to a doctor or a gynaecologist complaining of night sweats, they often relate it to a hormonal issue.

However, that is not the case. I have learned to manage my night sweats now — I eat an orange, walk a bit until my sweats come down and I can sleep again. I also go on a fruit-diet the next day!

Hormone Specific Therapies to Manage Fibromyalgia Pain

The hormone progesterone has been seen to have anti-inflammatory effects, and a recent study revealed an inverse relationship between testosterone levels and fibromyalgia.

A study conducted at Dartmouth Medical Centre had explored testosterone's ability to relieve some fibromyalgia symptoms. Many fibromyalgia patients outside India seem to be considering treating their pain symptoms with testosterone gel. However, I have not come across a testosterone hormone application. I believe that one should always investigate, understand, and then consider such treatments.

Hormonal intervention for treating hormonal imbalance is not a very good idea. That said, I would suggest that if at all one is considering this type of treatment, it has to be done only if it is the last resort – in times of emergency like massive bleeding or severe pain. Always remember, although hormone specific therapies can help modulate pain, it comes at a price. There are always the dangers of long-term side effects such as hot flashes, hair loss, sleep changes, etc.

The change in oestrogen and progesterone levels at different phases of a woman's life, such as puberty, pregnancy, and menopause, also play a crucial role in fibromyalgia pain.

Fibromyalgia - Puberty, Pregnancy, and Menopause

Puberty

Although commonly thought of as a condition that affects adults, fibromyalgia has been seen in children and adolescents.

Teen fibromyalgia is diagnosed in adolescent girls aged between 13 and 15. A 2013 study spoke about the promising approaches to juvenile fibromyalgia management [JFM] and noted that Cognitive Behavioural

Therapy [CBT] was a fairly promising mode of treatment for JFM.

Urinary tract infections are very common among young women; many are put under chronic antibiotic prophylactic therapy.

Symptoms

Frequent headaches, sleep disturbances, fatigue, stiffness, tightness, and frequent stomach aches are some of the major symptoms. The sleep disturbance might lead to cognitive impairment, and the child might find it difficult to remember academic information. This, in turn, results in her/him falling behind in school. Parents and teachers often misunderstand these symptoms. Thus, anxiety and depression are also commonly seen in teen fibromyalgia.

Diagnosis

Fibromyalgia is a difficult disease to diagnose in the first place. It becomes even more difficult in youngsters because when they complain of fatigue, headaches, and insomnia, they could be experiencing any one of several common illnesses.

Fibromyalgia is the last thing any doctor would suspect. A diagnosis of fibromyalgia in a child is made only after a long series of tests have ruled out other possible causes for the child's symptoms. In my experience, I have seen fibromyalgia in teenagers with autoimmune diseases,

Vasculitis, Ulcerative Colitis, and Crohn's disease. I have closely observed a friend's child suffering from Crohn's disease with pains all over his body.

As the diseases mentioned above also have fibromyalgia-like symptoms, it gets really difficult to diagnose this illness in children. Fibromyalgia is also sometimes seen in anaemic children.

A paediatric rheumatologist (a doctor who specialises in treating children with arthritis and other rheumatologic diseases) might be the go-to doctor in teen-fibromyalgia.

What Can Be Done?

Cognitive Behavioural Therapy [CBT] might help children with fibromyalgia identify as to what triggers their pain. Other behaviour-based approaches to treating fibromyalgia include muscle relaxation and stress-relieving techniques like meditation.

Exercise also goes a long way. Studies have shown that children with fibromyalgia who stay active feel less intense pain than those who are less active. That said, these children should also eat healthy and rest.

Pregnancy

A 2017 study investigated the frequency and most common symptoms of fibromyalgia among pregnant females and determined the impacts of the condition on the overall well-being. Among the 360 pregnant women studied, 37.7% were found to have fibromyalgia. It was also noticed that the painful areas were significantly higher in pregnant females with fibromyalgia. The lower back, upper leg, lower leg, and abdomen were the most affected sites.

Fibromyalgia symptoms such as pain, fatigue, and depression are very similar to those experienced by pregnant women. So, diagnosing fibromyalgia in pregnant ladies is even more difficult. Additionally, the added stress of having a baby could make things worse.Why are the painful areas significantly higher in pregnant women? Here's an explanation. Almost all pregnant women deal with sleep deprivation. We have learned in the previous chapters about the crucial role sleep plays in managing fibromyalgia pain.

Additionally, pregnancy brings about many hormonal changes, leg cramps, back pain, and many other physical aches that add to fibromyalgia pain. Yes, medications can help with the pain, but these medications may have side effects on the baby. Owing to all this, many women with fibromyalgia choose not to get pregnant at all.

On the other hand, even if a woman with fibromyalgia successfully gets through her pregnancy, the situation isn't free of concerns. Fibromyalgia sometimes flares up post-delivery, postpartum depression being the main contributor. In these cases, the new mother will have to go on medication to deal with her pain, which might adversely affect the baby through breastfeeding.

Remember, managing fibromyalgia during pregnancy, although difficult, is possible. Fibromyalgia should not stop you from planning a family. But it would be best if you spent some time learning about managing fibromyalgia during pregnancy.

Symptoms

Frequent mood changes heightened discomfort, fatigue, anxiety, depression, and other physical and emotional stress.

Diagnosis and Treatment

There's a tremendous increase in the number of hormones in a woman's body during pregnancy. Women with fibromyalgia are found to have heightened symptoms of pain, especially in the first three months.

Usually, fibromyalgia patients take prescribed painkillers and different medications to manage their pain. However, one has to worry in this case as medications might have side effects on the baby. So, the treatment for a pregnant woman with fibromyalgia may include massage, yoga, and meditation. Gentle stretching exercises can be practised under guidance as it helps strengthen the joints.

What Can Be Done?

1. Make sure to understand the risks and keep a check on all your symptoms.
2. Get some physical exercise under guidance. A daily walk can help a lot.

3. Always seek help.
4. The Journal of Pain Research has revealed that stretching can really help manage chronic pain during pregnancy.
5. Get enough sleep.

Menopause

Just like pregnant ladies, women with fibromyalgia going through menopause also have heightened emotions. Normal symptoms of menopause like hot flashes, leg pain, mood changes are at their peak. Most women often fail to realize that they are also dealing with fibromyalgia and menopause.

Most women are diagnosed with fibromyalgia, between the ages of 40 to 55, during menopause. Medical researchers believe symptoms noticed at this stage in a woman's life are most likely triggered by a decrease in oestrogen levels leading to anxiety, depression, and sleeplessness.

In my opinion, if the pain in any part of your body stays for more than a week, there's something wrong, and you need to consult a doctor. Women who confuse their aches for menopause, end up suffering from other side effects such as weight gain, sleep disturbances, and even depression.

PART C
DIAGNOSIS, TREATMENTS AND COST INVOLVED

Fibromyalgia is no more an 'unknown' disease. Many of us often suffer from stress and body aches. Most of us end up overworking in pursuit of a career. This increase in stress brings out many symptoms that mimic those of fibromyalgia. This makes the diagnosis very tricky. However, these days, if a patient complains of intense pain continuously for more than three or four months, doctors suspect fibromyalgia.

Medications such as antidepressants and anti-seizure drugs do help people manage their pain. However, none of these medications is free of side effects. Alternative therapies and recreational activities help patients destress and manage pain.

9
HOW EXPENSIVE IS IT TO TAKE CARE OF YOURSELF?

As we already know, there is no definite cure for fibromyalgia, yet. The treatment is symptomatic; drugs such as Amitriptyline, Duloxetine, Milnacipran or Pregabalin are usually prescribed to help control the symptoms. Along with traditional medications, a person with fibromyalgia is also advised to undergo physiotherapy, yoga therapy and many other alternative therapies.

Employing all these treatment techniques will surely burn a hole in your pockets. As there is no definite cure, you tend to try every treatment that can rid you of your pain and then stick to something that works.

Many of my patients suffering from fibromyalgia perceive different techniques and therapies as a waste of money. They find it completely pointless to spend money on treatments that cannot ensure relief. Well, this is true. Once you start, it does feel like there's no end to these therapy sessions. I went through it all. However, once you find what suits you the best, life becomes easier. For instance, today, I only practice yoga and physiotherapy [once every 15 days] — This is my only expense.

Does Life Insurance Cover Fibromyalgia?

Suffering from the chronic disease at a young age puts you in a tough spot, both personally and professionally. You often get into fights with your friends and family, which affects your professional life as well. Many even end up losing their jobs. This leads to an adverse effect on your financial situation.

Fibromyalgia has become a rather common disorder in recent times. So, in this day and age where hospital charges and other therapy and treatment costs shoot above the roof, it gets challenging for a middle-class person to deal with the disease. Many opt out of therapies due to their inability to afford it, and they end up dealing with intensified pain, which in turn takes a toll on their quality of life.

Decades ago, when fibromyalgia was not even considered an illness, applying for insurance might have been an issue. However, according to reports from 2019, fibromyalgia can be covered by critical illness insurance. While approving the insurance, the insurance companies often check if there are any negative effects of the medications you are taking. They also check if you consume alcohol, drugs and if you will be able to live a healthy life post the treatment. They will also want to know how long you have had fibromyalgia. The longer you have experienced the symptoms, the higher risk you are at of the side effects. In India, no outpatients are treated under medical insurance.

Can Early Diagnosis Help Cut Down the Expenses?

A study that evaluated the treatment initiation timing and healthcare costs among newly diagnosed fibromyalgia patients had revealed that the total healthcare costs were significantly lower among early-treated patients. Consuming fibromyalgia-related medications early on could actually be a cost-saving strategy.

A Holistic Approach to Treatment

Validating the patient's pain is where the treatment starts. A holistic approach to treatment includes medication to improve sleep, reduce pain, and address psychotherapeutic issues and behavioural management. The goal of treatment should be to improve the quality of life and productivity.

10 INDIVIDUAL THERAPIES

By now, we have understood that many factors come into play in the treatment of fibromyalgia. Regular workouts can help keep you flexible and help manage pain, to some extent. Various studies over the years have shown physiotherapy and Yoga as two most promising treatments used in fibromyalgia pain management. Additionally, aerobics, stretching, Tai chi, and other recreational activities also work miracles in the treatment of fibromyalgia.

Here's what you need to know about exercising. Always start slow. Do not push yourself. Know your limits and modify your workout schedule based on your physical and mental health. Additionally, do it under someone's guidance. Have an expert overseeing your exercise routine as injuries during workouts might add on to your fibromyalgia pain.

Now, read on as I talk about my personal experience with each therapy. I will describe how I dealt with my pain and how each of these therapies helped me. One thing I noticed while practicing these therapies was that whenever there's pain in a certain area, we tend to not perform that particular exercise. However, you must know that it is crucial for us to perform those stretches. If it is a long-standing spasm, a slow stretch in that particular muscle will help with the pain. So, even if it aches, make an effort and ensure that the muscle is completely stretched.

Physiotherapy

Physiotherapy is usually administered to help with the pain and stiffness of our muscles. This treatment helps build strength. As I mentioned in the earlier chapters, many advised me to consult a physiotherapist.

The first time I visited a physiotherapist was to release a particular muscle catch due to 'repetitive stress'. An ultrasonic release was performed and I must say, releasing the knots with ultrasound therapy gave me instant relief. However, one thing about physiotherapy is that you have to do it regularly.

For example, if I discontinued ultrasound therapy for two consecutive days, my pain would take a turn for the worse.

I want to talk about the importance of releasing muscle knots here. These knots are the primary reason for pain. Also known as the myofascial trigger points, these muscle knots are bump-like areas of muscle that ache when you touch them.

These are common in places where there are repetitive stress and more nerve endings—calf muscles, lower back, shins, shoulders, and neck are some of the spots where muscle knots generally occur. These are hard and quite sensitive. In fibromyalgia, there are multiple knots in the areas mentioned above.

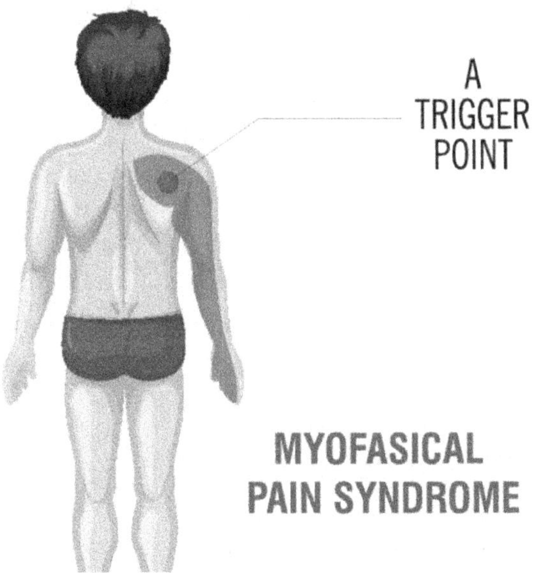

Now, how are these muscle knots caused? Here's an explanation.

1. Sedentary Lifestyle:

This is the main culprit. Being idle all day with no body movement whatsoever might cause muscle knots.

2. Over-Stressing or Injury to The Muscles:

When there's excessive pressure on muscles, muscle knots are pretty common.

3. Dehydration and Bad Eating Habits:

By keeping your body hydrated, you can defend your body against many problems. Drinking lots of water prevents chemical imbalances in the muscle, thus avoiding knots.

4. Sitting in A Poor Posture for A Long Time:

This is another major contributor to muscle knot. Correct posture puts the least amount of strain on your muscles and joints.

5. Stress

Stress also causes muscle knots. Chronic stress on our muscles creates micro-tearing of muscle tissue, which creates scar tissue and knots.

High-Risk Category:

Muscle knots are quite common. However, there are a few specific factors that might increase the chances of developing muscles knots.

Ageing is first on the list. If someone is already suffering from a chronic disorder, they are also at a higher risk of getting muscle knots. People suffering from fibromyalgia are commonly diagnosed with muscle knots.

Fact: Once muscle knots are released, the muscles can be maintained in good condition using Yoga, stretch therapy or any other low metabolic exercises.

Coming back to my physiotherapy journey, I continued the therapy with one of the best practitioners in town. I was undergoing treatment every alternate day as the pain was severe. Around the same time, I also learnt about chiropractors. I was told that a good chiropractor could relieve me of pain. I realised mechanical problems in muscles could affect the skeletal system.

Chiropractic care primarily focuses on disorders of the musculoskeletal and nervous systems. Interestingly enough, although I was fully aware that a disease like fibromyalgia had no cure, I gave in and told myself that proper chiropractic treatment might save me and take me out of my misery!

There is not much difference between a physiotherapy and chiropractic treatment, except for the mode of treatment. While physiotherapists help with pain management and improved mobility, chiropractors focus on aligning parts of the body; they focus on the affected areas. However, pain-management and pain relief are the primary goals of both these techniques.

I wanted to consult the best chiropractor in the world. As per my research and based on the information I collected from other sources, the best ones were in the USA. Following this, I flew to New York in 2011 and consulted a chiropractor for eight days in a row. I stayed for a total of 15 days in New York.

I explained my situation to the chiropractor and told him about the specific areas where the pain was severe. I was administered the push-pull therapy.

This is how push-pull therapy works: There are movable tables. The experts manually put pressure on the joints, stretch it and then pull them back to its position. This therapy helps stabilise each joint. In fact, the results were so promising that I also discussed it with my physiotherapist and Yoga therapist back home. The chiropractor also taught me some exercises which not just helped me with the pain, but also strengthened my tendons[muscles].

After about two weeks of treatment in New York, I flew back to India sometime in October. I was delighted with the progress I had made. Since I felt okay, I got back to my practice and resumed my work at the hospital. I was so busy that I ended up overworking during November.

As expected, due to all the overwork and overstress I put my body through, I started experiencing pain again; and this time, it was intolerable. It was worse because this time, it hit me hard emotionally. I had spent so much time and energy, going all the way to New York, and I was happy about my treatment. I just did not expect my pain to come back, not so soon!

So, if I had stayed home for a long time after my chiropractic treatment, do you think the treatment would have worked? Well, I don't know. It might have, or it might have not. I am a surgeon, and I had to get back to work at some point. Let's assume the patient is a housewife. Now, a homemaker can't just sit idle for months together, right? As they say, an empty mind is a devil's workshop. The idler you are, the more you end up thinking about your illness. So, I don't regret getting back to work. In fact, I think my work gave me the strength to fight my illness.

How Exactly Does Physiotherapy Help Fibromyalgia?

Physiotherapy reduces stiffness and fatigue. A physiotherapist can help you with pain management, pain-relief and also with a range of motion exercises. This is exactly what you require in case of fibromyalgia.

Passive and active treatments are the two types of treatments administered in physiotherapy. While passive treatment refers to massage, active treatments refer to flexibility exercises. Although physiotherapy does not provide a long-term cure, it sure helps you identify the area of pain, and this is a big help in case of fibromyalgia.

Massage Therapy

This therapy involves the moving of muscles and soft tissues. People opt for massage therapy hoping for relaxation, and a good massage can give you just that. It can also help reduce heart rate, destress your muscles, and increase the flow of blood in your body.

Many with fibromyalgia prefer massage therapy as it helps them relieve stress, both physically and mentally. A 2014 study conducted to evaluate the benefits of massage therapy for patients with fibromyalgia had revealed that massage therapy over five weeks had beneficial effects on improving pain, anxiety, and depression. Massage therapy helped me. The massage therapist released many knots in my right shoulder, upper right and lower back areas.

However, I also must tell you that massage therapy has its side effects. Although this therapy enhances blood flow and helps the blood absorb more nutrients and remove toxins, there's a slight crushing of muscles during the process; it can bring temporary discomfort and increase inflammation. Hence, I used to take paracetamol and other pain medications during my massage therapy sessions. Also, I underwent another type of therapy called 'Shiatsu'; it is a very gentle and sublime massage technique that has origins in Japan and dates back to around 2,500 years ago.

Shiatsu helps deal with migraines, hormonal issues like PMS, PTSD, sleep deprivation and even depression. In fibromyalgia, since the person deals with many emotional sufferings, shiatsu could be of great help to calm an overactive mind.

How Exactly Does Massage Therapy Help the Fibromyalgia?

Massage therapy helps in alleviating anxiety, depression, and sleep disturbance. Even if it provides only short-term relief, it means to a lot to the patient. Myofascial release and Connective Tissue Massage[CTM] are among the two main types of massage therapies.

Myofascial Release:

This type of release helps the patient with muscle pain and stiffness by relaxing contracted muscles. This release also helps improve blood flow.

Connective Tissue Massage [CTM]

CTM is a method of applying firm pressure and massaging the deeper layers of the skin. This type of release helps reduce muscle tension and chronic pains.

Yoga Therapy

Yoga therapy is very promising. It involves the use of various asanas [poses], breathing exercises [pranayama] and meditation. It helps with the overall development of mind and body. Yoga helps in alleviating anxiety and depression. In fact, a 2020 study had demonstrated a reduction in muscle fatigue and improvement in the quality of life and sleep in fibromyalgia patients using Yoga therapy.

I had tried Yoga back in 2012, but the tutor had me do all the asanas so fast that I ended up experiencing heightened pain. After that incident, I never really took to it again. However, in the beginning of 2014, when I had tried almost all treatments, and nothing helped substantially, many advised me to give Yoga another try. I made up my mind and tried Yoga with another therapist.

This time, I asked my therapist to go at a slow pace and luckily, she agreed.

There are two types of Yoga therapy – Dynamic and Power. I was comfortable with dynamic Yoga. I used to practice Yoga for one straight hour every day, early in the morning, and the results were quite promising; I noticed these changes in just a couple of weeks.

Practising Yoga helped me identify my pain areas. Additionally, I could feel the pain and the active knots in my body, a few months after I started practising Yoga. This actually helped me a lot as I could point out the pain areas and the active knots to my physiotherapist or a massage therapist, who then helped me by releasing those knots. Among all the therapies that we discussed, Yoga has helped me the most. I would recommend everyone reading this book to start practising Yoga. Suppose you are already doing so, congratulations. If not, start right away!

How Does Yoga Help Fibromyalgia?

As I mentioned earlier, the only therapy that I have been practising for a long time now is Yoga. Yoga reduces stress, calms you down and as we know, stress is one of the main culprits in fibromyalgia.

A condition like fibromyalgia needs to be treated with great care. The pain can be triggered at any time, and it is hard to say what causes the pain. For something so vague, Yoga is the best treatment. It treats your entire body and helps heal from within.

As Yoga is usually combined with breathing exercises [pranayama], it is an added advantage. Pranayama stimulates the parasympathetic nervous system; deep breathing helps deal with intense pain and anxiety.

Many studies over the years have confirmed Yoga's positive impact on the quality of life in patients who have fibromyalgia. Additionally, we also learnt about the hormonal effects on fibromyalgia and the heightened pain during periods. It is said that a lot of Yoga poses help in correcting hormonal imbalance. The butterfly asana [Baddha Konasana], for example, is very good for the uterus. So, Yoga can help correct your hormonal balance, giving fibromyalgia patients some relief during their menstrual cycle.

Researchers say that practising Yoga might also rewire the central system's response to pain signals. A study conducted at Oregon Health &Science University revealed that Yoga assists in combating several serious fibromyalgia symptoms including pain, fatigue, stiffness, poor sleep, depression, poor memory, anxiety and poor balance.

Belief is also an important element. While practising Yoga, tell yourself that you are going to be okay and that practising Yoga will help you heal. In this section, I'm sharing with you all the important asanas that I practised, and I am practising even today. Many Yoga poses can potentially benefit a person with fibromyalgia, but here are some asanas that I personally recommend.

Surya Namaskar

It is usually performed in the morning. As the name suggests, this asana is perceived as a salute to Lord Surya.

Surya namaskar has many benefits. It increases cardiac activity, lengthens the spine, stretches the muscles, improves self-awareness and flexibility, relieves fatigue, stiffness, and body pain and builds stamina.

The patients suffering from fibromyalgia have a lot of negative energy around them. Practising Surya Namaskar every day brings positive energy, increases alertness, and brings more confidence.

Remember one thing, Surya namaskar should always be practised by following the right breathing techniques; only then will you receive the maximum benefits. The coordination between the two is also necessary for easy movement.

Trikonasana [Triangle Pose]

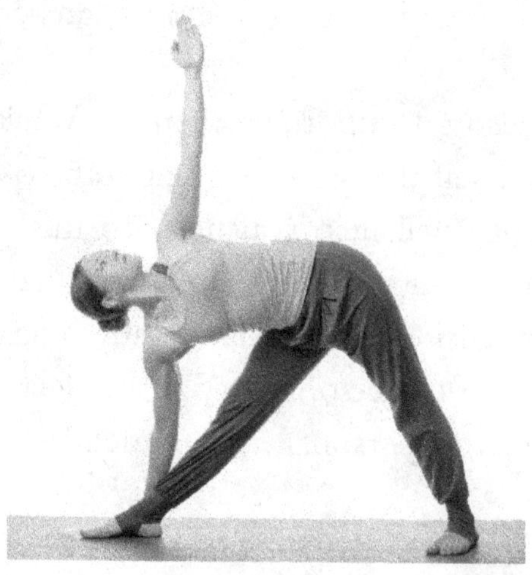

Trikonasana strengthens the rib-cage, and the pelvis area along with legs, knees, ankles, arms and chest. These lateral stretches helps in releasing the paraspinal muscles and reduces the stiffness in the abdominal wall. This asana helps women with their menstrual and menopause problems as well.

Dhanurasana [Bow Pose]

Dhanurasana helps a lot with abdominal pain. The asana looks like a bow, hence the name. This pose provides internal organs with an excellent and powerful massage.

This asana also has other health benefits as it treats asthma, helps weight loss, increases flexibility, and strengthens the lower back. It also helps take control of your emotions, manage diabetes and other hormonal issues.

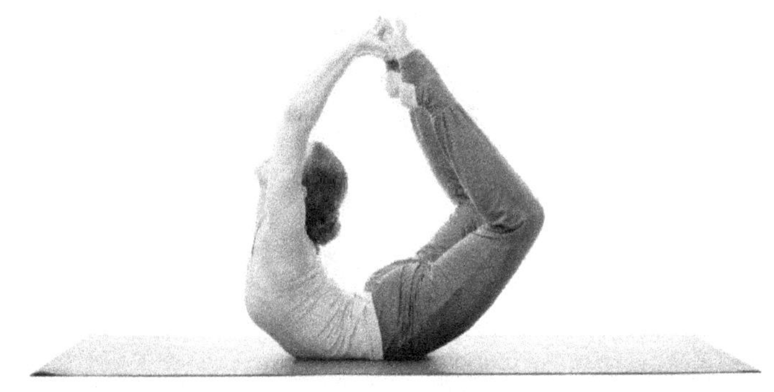

Vrkshasana [Tree Pose]

Vrksasana is another very beneficial asana that is popularly known for increasing concentration. This asana helps prevent knots in the anterior aspect of the thigh. Although these knots can be released with therapies, in my case, they usually came back whenever I walked a lot. So, practising Vrkshasana helped me get rid of the knots. Vrkshasana also helps in balancing the functions of the large intestines and adrenals. It also helped my neuro-muscular coordination.

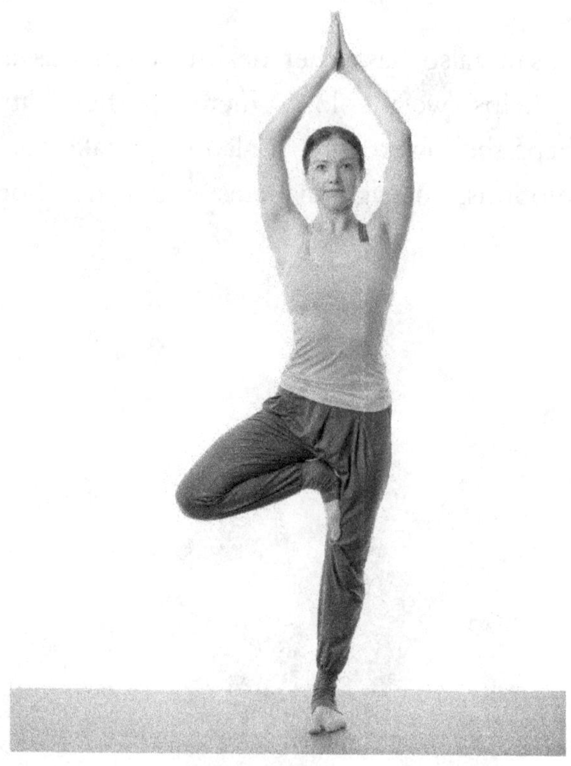

Balasana [Child's Pose]

Child's pose is the best asana to practice if you are suffering from too much anxiety. It calms down your nerves and helps you reflect on your thoughts. This asana also facilitates better blood circulation, which in turn helps with migraines and other headaches. Balasana can help with high blood pressure, irritable bowel syndrome and anxiety, which are some of the major issues in fibromyalgia.

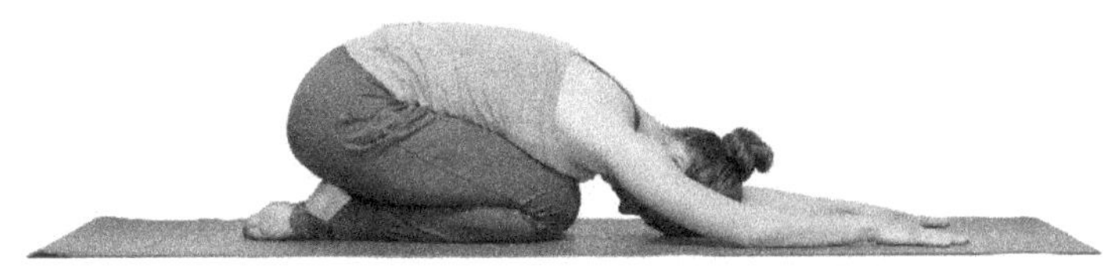

Other Approaches for Fibromyalgia

Tai chi is another promising practice that helps relieve fibromyalgia pain. Tai chi also includes several breathing exercises.

Steroid Therapy

Steroids are usually injected to treat inflammation. However, a steroid injected directly into a trigger point has not always been successful. There are no studies that support the success of steroid therapy in fibromyalgia patients.

Although I was convinced about steroid therapy, initially, I agreed to get it done on one of my knots. Steroids were injected into one of my knots in the trapezius muscle – one of the largest knots in the body which did not respond to ultrasound, massage and even Yoga therapy. Surprisingly, steroid therapy helped me with that knot. I do not take it anymore, but if someone is suffering from too many rigid knots in their body, I'd suggest them to give steroid therapy a try.

11
DIET

The food that we consume in the present day is not entirely healthy. There are pesticide residues in fruits and vegetables, which can have acute and chronic health effects. Thus, it is vital that we take the utmost care of

ayuh-sattva-balarogya-sukha-priti-vivardhanah rasyah snigdhah
sthira hrdya aharah sattvika-priyah
katv-amla-lavanaty-usna-tiksna-ruksa-vidahinah ahara
rajasasyesta duhkha-sokamaya-pradah
yata-yamam gata-rasam puti paryusitam ca yat ucchistam api
camedhyam
bhojanam tamasa-priyam

As mentioned on asitis.com: Foods in the mode of goodness increase the duration of life, purify one's existence and give strength, health, happiness and satisfaction. Such nourishing foods are sweet, juicy, fattening and palatable. Foods that are too bitter, too sour, salty, pungent, dry and hot, are liked by people in the modes of passion. Such foods cause pain, distress, and disease. Food cooked more than three hours before being eaten, which is tasteless, stale, putrid, decomposed and unclean, is food liked by people in the mode of ignorance.[3]

what we eat when we eat and how we eat.

Further, we are often advised to consume an antioxidant diet — Antioxidant diet helps us fight against heart disease, cancer, and many other diseases. However, the food that we consume daily, especially proteins, is known to produce more oxidants.

Sometimes, we unknowingly end up consuming food that we might be intolerant or allergic to — This leads to a reaction in the gut, which causes damage and results in the formation of oxidants (toxins). These toxins get into our bodies and become a part of our circulation, muscles, and affect digestion. This further leads to fatigue, bloating, and muscular pain. In fact, this food intolerance may be the first sign of autoimmune disease.

A plant-based diet is the best source of antioxidants. A 2001 study had revealed that a raw vegetarian diet helped alleviate fibromyalgia symptoms. A vegetarian diet helps remove the toxins accumulated in the cells and boosts the functioning of muscle fibre activity in fibromyalgia.

Here's another intriguing fact. It has been proven repeatedly that fibromyalgia can be effectively dealt with if a few changes are made in the patient's dietary habits. For instance, fibromyalgia patients are often seen to be lactose intolerant. The dairy products contain saturated fat, and excessive intake of saturated fats causes inflammation and pain.

So, if the patient cuts down on all dairy products, it might help manage the pain. Various studies over the years have established that food allergy is one of the significant conditions associated with fibromyalgia.

Go Vegetarian!

Believe it or not, switching to a plant-based diet is the best way to get your health back on track. Going vegetarian improves the health of your gut and reduces inflammation. It also helps boost your immune system. The fibre from a plant-based diet can lower cholesterol and stabilize blood sugar. It also facilitates good bowel management. Many people all over the world are trying to make the switch in recent years.

Consuming a plateful that includes plenty of fresh fruits and vegetables, whole grains, and healthy fats may help manage inflammation.

The importance of a balanced diet has been taught to us since our school days; too much protein can increase inflammation in your body, and excess carbohydrate intake might lead to weight gain, poor metabolic health, and an increased risk of heart disease.

I could not follow a good diet due to my busy schedule; I did not restrict myself when it came to eating. However, upon learning about the different effects food allergy has on fibromyalgia pain, I made it a point to control my erratic dietary habits.

In 2017, as suggested by a patient of mine, I underwent a test that pointed out the food items I was allergic to. The results showed that I was allergic to egg, milk, cornflour, gluten flax seeds, and many other cereal kinds.

As I'm a vegetarian, our primary source of nutrition includes pulses, and to my bad luck, I was allergic to those. I was not even allowed to eat Idli and Dosa, as they are made of Urad dal. I switched to a rice-based diet, vegetables, and fruits.

Fibromyalgia can make you feel tired and worn out very soon. So, make sure to consume food that gives you a lot of energy. Sweets are a quick sugar boost, but unhealthy in the long run.

Instead of these instant energy boosters, opt for fruits and other food items low in added sugars. Weight loss decreases inflammation and eases the burden on your muscles and joints.

What can I Eat, Then?

1. **Almonds and Other Dry Fruits**:

The craving for something to munch on while working is quite common. I suggest you keep some almonds and other dry fruits by your side. Junk food items have no health benefits, whereas dry fruits provide energy and build stamina.

2. **Broccoli**

Broccoli is high in many nutrients, including fibre, vitamin C, vitamin K, iron, and potassium. It is also a good source of protein. Steamed broccoli is highly recommended.

3. Beans and Lentils

Beans and lentils are low in fat content and provide us with loads of Vitamin B, K, and magnesium content. For vegetarians, legumes can be the best substitute for meat.

Lentils also aid in weight loss. As we all know, the fibre contents help in digestion. They are also high in antioxidants.

4. Oatmeal and Barley

Oats and Barley help lower the cholesterol level, preventing type 2 diabetes and other heart-related diseases.

5. Leafy Greens

Leafy greens are rich in vitamins A, B, C, E, and K and iron; they provide the energy required for the body to function every day.

6. Herbs and Spices

Herbs and spices are rich in antioxidants, and antioxidants help reduce inflammation. Turmeric, bay leaves, cinnamon, ginger, cumin, fennel, garlic, and cloves are usually used in cooking every day. Additionally, turmeric has also been proven to be useful in treating people with rheumatoid arthritis.

What Shouldn't I Eat?

1. Avoid Artificial Sweeteners and Limit Sugars

For general good health, avoid artificial sweeteners. Minimize the amount of sugar in your diet as high sugar leads to a number of inflammatory diseases.

2. Avoid Food That Triggers Inflammation.

- Gluten-containing foods
- Food additives or food chemicals
- Excitotoxins, such as MSG
- Saturated fats and trans fats
- Refined starches
- Foods with added sugar
- Additives - Food additives called excitotoxins may worsen some of the symptoms of fibromyalgia.

3. Avoid Alcohol

Refrain from alcohol and other substances when you are on medication. Although some people with fibromyalgia had reported comfort when they had a few drinks, remember, the pain always comes back once the effect wears off. Moreover, alcohol can affect your hormones.

Learn About the Body's Reaction to Certain Foods

If food appears to trigger symptoms in an individual, eliminating the food for several weeks is an excellent way to determine its impact. Keeping a detailed food log to track symptoms when the food is removed and added back may also be helpful.

Reducing sugar and sugary foods can have an additional benefit; it can help the individual overcome a craving for sweets in the long term. The doctor can be a useful resource on food sensitivities and should be informed of problems encountered with different foods and ingredients. In some cases, the doctor may suggest testing for food sensitivities or allergies to narrow the list of potentially allergic foods.

Keep a Food Diary

Whenever you feel discomfort after consuming a meal, write down what you ate, and note down the sufferings and allergies you are going through. The next time you crave for that food, you will stop yourself from eating that particular food. Similarly, make a note of vegetables that help you and consume more of them.

Food Items Rich in Antioxidants:

1. Eat eight to nine servings of fruits and vegetables per day: Eating various colourful fruits and vegetables can ensure the most fantastic range of nutrients. Foods that are incredibly rich in nutrients include broccoli and berries.
2. Choose whole grains: Whole-grain foods include Barley, buckwheat, oats, quinoa, brown rice, rye, wheat, and spelling These foods provide vitamins, protein, and fibre.
3. Choose healthful oils: Olive oil is the right choice.

Do Nightshade Vegetables Increase Fibromyalgia Pain?

Nightshade vegetables include potatoes, peppers, eggplant, and tomatoes. All of them contain a toxin known as solanine that can increase inflammation in the joints and may increase pain in fibromyalgia patients.

Will Changing the Diet Really Help One Cope with Fibromyalgia?

Yes, it definitely will. Many patients who have made the necessary changes in their dietary habits are now leading a healthy life. Although dietary changes can't be considered a treatment for fibromyalgia, they act as a helping hand in managing the symptoms.

Here Are A Few Changes That I Made in My Diet:

- Instead of making *Rotis* [Indian bread] out of wheat, I use jawar, rice, and millet.
- Instead of making *upma* out of broken wheat, I use broken millet and broken jawar.
- I also stopped eating cake and all other bakery items. Instead, I use rice/jawar flour to make dry snacks.
- I eat fruits three times a day.
- I also take multivitamins and omega 3 fatty acids to detoxify oxidants.

12
IS DIAGNOSIS IMPORTANT?

Unlike the diagnosis of other diseases, in fibromyalgia, the patient plays a vital role. Since there is no particular test, the diagnosis entirely depends on the patient's description of pain. It is essential that the patient opens up to the physician. In my case, I kept going in for several diagnoses; I was investigating the condition myself; hence I went in for multiple diagnoses. However, I was always met with a vague conclusion. There was no clarity about my condition whatsoever.

In many such situations, when the diagnosis isn't clear after multiple attempts, the patients are treated based on the most common condition and then observed. My investigations pointed towards inflammatory and autoimmune diseases. However, there also seemed to be an association with a few viral infections, especially RNA viruses, because fibromyalgia usually starts as a muscular/joint pain. In my view, the below-mentioned are the known investigations involved in the diagnosis of fibromyalgia.

1. Routine investigation
2. Viral markers
3. Nonspecific investigations for inflammation
4. Evaluation for tuberculosis
5. Specific investigations once the diagnosis is heading in a specific direction – Many patients often end up getting a colonoscopy and endoscopy done.

Let's understand the step-by-step process of diagnosis in fibromyalgia. Widespread pain lasting over a span of three months or more should be your first clue. Be it any pain, and if it is prolonged for more than three-four months, there is definitely an underlying condition. Additionally, if the patient also suffers from tenderness, stiffness, fatigue, insomnia, and other cognitive difficulties, the situation needs to be addressed immediately. However, these symptoms might be pointing to any other disorder. So, how exactly is the diagnosis made? And how does it help the situation? Let's dig a little deeper.

The American College of Rheumatologist [ACR] had laid down a set of guidelines way back in 1990, which helped in the diagnosis of fibromyalgia. It was based on tenderness in at least 11 out of 18 tender points in our body [Neck, Arms, Shoulders, Back, Chest, Abdomen,

Thighs, Pelvis among others], otherwise known as widespread body pain index[WPI].

Although this method proved to be successful in the initial years, it was later observed that since the pain comes and goes and shifts to different areas in fibromyalgia, the disorder could not be confirmed based on the tender points alone. Hence, the criteria were updated in 2010, wherein the severity of the symptom was taken into consideration rather than the WPI. In this updated version of guidelines, other factors like the cognitive symptoms, sleep and fatigue were also monitored.

Additionally, the National Fibromyalgia and Chronic Pain Association had concluded around the same time that prolonged axial skeletal pain (cervical spine, anterior chest, thoracic spine or low back pain) might also be pointing towards fibromyalgia.

Although both the methods did not completely prove to be useful, something productive did come out of them. A Widespread Pain Index (WPI) and Symptom Severity (SS) scale made way for a 42-question symptom questionnaire that helped rule out other disorders, leading to an accurate fibromyalgia diagnosis—The National Fibromyalgia & Chronic Pain Association stood by this.

At the moment, the following three points are widely used by physicians across the world to diagnose fibromyalgia.

- How widespread is the pain and how severe is it?
- Has it been prolonged for more than three months?

- Medical history and other possible explanations for their sufferings.

The first step in diagnosing fibromyalgia is ruling out the other conditions. Rheumatoid arthritis, Lupus, Hypothyroidism, are some of the "copycats" as noted by the ACR. In my view, anyone who suffers from prolonged joint pain should first consult a rheumatologist.

Once the rheumatologist rules out other arthritic conditions and confirms fibromyalgia, you can return to your primary physician and manage your condition. Conditions that can be ruled out:

- Hypothyroidism
- Addison's disease
- Hyperparathyroidism
- Lupus
- Lyme disease
- Multiple sclerosis (MS)
- Post-traumatic stress disorder (PTSD)
- Rheumatoid arthritis
- Scleroderma

A study conducted in 2010 has concluded that delay in the diagnosis of fibromyalgia only worsens the condition. The survey answered by 800 patients with fibromyalgia from eight countries concluded that this condition had a notable impact on their quality of life and that the current treatment options were not satisfactory. Remember to write down all your symptoms as and when you experience them. As fibromyalgia entails cognitive difficulties as well, you do not want to miss out on any symptom.

Before I wrap up this chapter, I would like to emphasise the importance of diet. We spoke extensively about diet in the previous chapter. Even today, after almost a decade of suffering from fibromyalgia, I experience night sweats, indigestion, dryness of mouth and eyes whenever I consume egg, any type of lentils, milk and other dairy products.

In my opinion, the toxins produced due to the antigen and antibody reaction inside my body damages my glandular system; there must be some antigen/antibody connection to the glandular system. It's 2021, and there are still no definite answers to fibromyalgia. Instead of waiting to be diagnosed or treated for fibromyalgia, I'd recommend everyone to start a plant-based and fruit-based diet the moment they begin experiencing the symptoms mentioned in the previous chapters. Prevention is always better than cure.

13
FAMILY AND FRIENDS

Let us now talk about the importance of family and friends in the life of a patient dealing with fibromyalgia. There are numerous factors that family and friends have to keep in mind. Firstly, assure the patient that it's all going to okay. Tell the patient that it is fine if she wants to stay by herself and not mingle. Acknowledge the fact that she is in pain and provide her with emotional support. Friends and family play a crucial role in the patient's recovery.

You can contribute a ton just by understanding the patient's condition. One should always focus on making the patient feel comfortable in her own skin. Since the patients have many limitations because of their condition, help them adapt to their new routine.

I'm writing this chapter to acknowledge and thank all of my family members and friends who have prayed for my well-being and helped me recover. My husband,

Rajaneesh, was my pillar of strength. He completely understood what I was going through and stood by me throughout my journey. In fact, on the days that I slept well, I could see the relief on his face the next morning!

My daughter was a teenager when I was going through all this. If there's anything I regret in my life, it is the time that I could not spend with her. I was away from her for nearly four years. However, I am glad that my husband and in-laws were there for her. My husband always made it a point to spend time with her. My mother-in-law had me in her prayers.

I was always on edge at home, given my condition. There would often be heightened disturbance in the family due to my unpredictable behaviour and extreme health situation. However, none of my family members gave up on me. I would like to thank them for all their support.

I am blessed to have a few exceptional friends in my life. They provided me with the strength that I needed. In fact, it was during this time that I realised who my actual friends were. As all of them had seen me during my healthier days, none of them could believe what I was going through.

The best thing that happened to me amid all this was that no one judged me—I am thankful for that.

On the whole, it has been one hell of a journey. I have experienced the best and the worst. There were many days when I gave up hope. If I am alive and have successfully gotten back to my old self today, it is firstly because of my determination and secondly, and most importantly, because of the support I received from my family and friends.

Last but definitely not least, I would like to thank all my doctors. They played a significant role in guiding me; I was fortunate enough to be treated by the best doctors. All of them were supportive in their own ways. I was treated in a dignified, friendly manner. They believed in my research and the knowledge I had about my condition. Here are a few heartfelt notes about me and my life written by a few people very close to my heart. Please read on.

Rajaneesh
Husband

Fibromyalgia was an alien word back in 2009. Nanda was in a long and dark tunnel trapped in muscle fatigue, body ache, breathlessness, and mood swings. Expert medical consultations and several tests did not lead to any diagnosis. Lost in the labyrinth, Nanda eventually realized it was up to her to confront this demon of a disease and figure out ways to deal with it. She read up extensive medical literature, changed the diet and adjusted work, and eventually swam out to the shore from deep sea. It was a very difficult time for all of us.

Nikita
Daughter

The first time I was terrified was when we were in Goa on vacation, and my mother woke up in the middle of the night, screaming with pain. It was horrifying and concerning because no matter how much work she had at the hospital, she would always tend to the family at the end of the day. No matter how tired she was, we could approach her any time of the day, and she would listen to us.

Mother's positive energy was contagious. She always lit up her surroundings with her cheerful personality. But fibromyalgia consumed her. My warm and caring mother became aloof and dismissive. I don't know what she exactly went through, but I know that her body pain was so intense that it clouded who she really was. After suffering quite a bit, my mother found every ounce of strength she had left and fought fibromyalgia like a champion. Once she was cured, my adorable mother was back to pestering me and caring for all my needs.

Bala Deshpande

I met Dr. Nanda in a professional capacity nearly a decade ago. Since both of us stayed in different cities and had no frequent meetings or common business agendas, we never really got to meet often. However, Nanda is one of my closest friends, and I deeply cherish the bond we both share. While Nanda is a unique combination of intelligence and a child-like innocence in worldly matters, she is also a doctor with great expertise in her field. Happy to write about her!

I must bring up a strange coincidence that sealed our bond of trust and friendship. The very first long conversation I had with Nanda was on my health. I am an avid traveller, but sometimes visiting different places creates great havoc on my stomach, my digestion, and other related discomforts.

Nanda launched herself into finding out the best way to reduce my distress. She won me over with her dogged determination, her extensive research, and the simple fact that she cared enough.

The coincidence I am referring to is that a few years later, Nanda herself became a victim of several physical symptoms. I could see that whatever she was fighting affected her joie-de-vivre and led to visible changes in her personality. It was tough to see her struggle; however, unlike her, I could only play a sympathetic friend's role and could not help or guide her to fight this unknown health enemy.

Then one fine day, the spirit of never-say-die retook Nanda, and she clawed back to normalcy inch by inch. She has come out of this battle not just successfully but as a stronger, wiser person. Kudos to her.

I am sure that as time goes by, Nanda will develop into a persona who will be able to influence millions of people and bring about a positive impact and change.

Dr. B G Dharmanand

When I saw Dr. Nanda as a patient, she was a young surgeon on her way up in the surgical field, which, by the way, is a stronghold of male surgeons. Her unexpected illness and mysterious pains had started putting a spoke in her journey.

The only role I played here was to confirm the diagnosis and provide her with pharmaceutical and non-pharmaceutical measures. The rest was all Nanda.

She did her own research and tried many modalities before synthesizing an excellent way of managing her illness. Full credits to Dr. Nanda!

Now, after many years, I see her as a champion who found her own ways to overcome this complex illness. I wish her all the luck with this book.

I'm sure it will help thousands of patients on their path to recovery.

Dr. Shivanna

Despite working with Dr. Nanda for more than two years, I was unaware of the pains she was going through, until the day Dr. Nanda herself told me about her sufferings. Being a practising chronic pain specialist and acupuncture specialist, Dr. Nanda and I worked together and chalked out an acupuncture regime to release the muscle knots; this helped her immensely.

I spoke to Dr. Nanda after a long gap, and I was delighted to know that she was writing a book on her journey, with the sole intention of helping other fibromyalgia patients. That's the Nanda I knew—always willing to help others and concerned of others' well-being. I wish her all the luck.

Meena Kodandaram

There are no coincidences in life. We meet the right people at the right time, who end up changing our whole course of life. And some of them become friends for life! It was during one summer party that I met this elegant lady, and she literally changed my life! The bond that I share with her is beyond words. She has been my support system throughout.

My father was diagnosed with stage 4 lung cancer. When she learned about this, despite her busy work schedule, family, and hundreds of other extracurricular activities, Nanda made time and spoke to me about my father's condition.

She volunteered to do her research into the illness and guided me through one of the most challenging times of my life. While being a pillar of strength for me, she fought her own battle with food allergy and wide-spread body pains. I am amazed at how she managed to juggle through it all.

A few months ago, I had the diagnosis of disc herniation with degenerative disc disease. My active life came to a standstill because of muscle weakness, spasms, and pain. Again, it was Nanda who held my hand.

While it seemed like the doctors prescribed all the pain killers available at the pharmacy, Nanda took a step back and suggested consuming nutritious food instead. She taught me the importance of massages, yoga, nutrition, and she made sure that I could control my dependence on pain killers by observing what I ate.

I will always be indebted to her for helping me live a near-normal life. I am truly blessed to have her in my life as my doctor, conscience, and best friend.

Pushpalatha

Nanda and I became close friends the very first time we met. There was an instant spark between us, and I think that might have been the case because I resembled her sister. We have known each other for many years now.

Talking about Nanda, well, she is so many things. She's an active, intelligent, beautiful lady who is very efficient in whatever she does. I admire her for her courage and determination.

Nanda is also a big-time foodie. She always used to walk into our house, sit down with us and munch on home-cooked food and snacks. However, as days passed, I was surprised to see her complain about indigestion and other stomach/gut related discomfort.

As far as I knew, she had always been a healthy person. I later realized that she was allergic to certain kinds of food items. She had also started to put on weight.

I'm sure she had noticed all these changes, but she never mentioned anything to me, and neither did I ask her about anything.

Even though I would stop her from eating the food items she was allergic to, she would end up eating it anyway and would assure me that everything would be fine if she went home and took her medicine.

I gradually started hiding the snacks as soon as I heard her coming in because I did not want her to get tempted and suffer the consequences.

However, off late, I have noticed that she has developed some kind of food control in her routine. She says no to specific snacks even if I offer it to her.

This is a new version of Nanda. Such a drastic change! Now, Nanda eats healthy food and has excellent control over her food habits. I'm thrilled to see Nanda recovering and getting back to her old self.

Dr. Sudhir Borgonha

I have had the good fortune of knowing Nanda as a friend for over ten years. She is a remarkable person, a thorough professional, and a friend who you can count on always!

Like all of us, Nanda has had her own challenges. One of them is the onset of a varied set of symptoms that specialists struggled to diagnose. A spectrum of tests, a battery of specialists, trying multiple therapeutic approaches, and a lot of research went into trying to narrow down a diagnosis.

I believe it was the spirit that Nanda echoes, unflailing courage to seek an answer and then apply all her strength to overcome it. To me, that focus, that conviction, that drive when the rest of the world is lost, is courage. During those tumultuous times, she had the courage to seek all forms of support, including mental health, a taboo subject for a successful medical professional.

Dr. Sumitha Shankar

I have seen Dr. Nanda come out of her struggles with health issues in connection with fibromyalgia and other emotional components related to it. With her deep, rich understanding and disciplined nutritional aspects, she overcame most of her health problems. Overall, I would say she is very caring, articulative, and approachable. These qualities have been significant contributors not only in healing herself but also the people around her.

One such bold example I have noticed is her relationship with her daughter, which has grown into mutual respect and friendship, enabling her daughter to be a fine grown-up, mature adult.

Ruchika Dawar

I have known Dr. Nanda for over three years now. She is a wonderful lady with a heart of gold, and her knowledge about every subject is something that I admire.

Nanda is a go-getter. If she sets her mind to something, she will accomplish it come what may. Despite her hectic schedule and health issue of fibromyalgia, she made sure to some time out every day for her fitness and yoga sessions.

Even today, Dr. Nanda practices deep breathing and various other pranayama techniques. We perform classical hatha yoga, holding each posture for a little longer duration to stretch every muscle.

Some of the critical asanas that are practised during our sessions are *Uttanasana, Parvatasana, Balasana, Bhujangasana, Baddha Konasana, Virabhadrasana,* and *Vrikshasana*—All these help stretch the body well.

During these practice sessions, we do face a few challenges like muscle spasm; however, Nanda is so determined that she does not let anything come in the way of her practice. That's when deep breathing plays a crucial role.

She is also very particular about her diet and ensures that she eats a dairy-free, gluten-free diet. She also includes a lot of fresh fruits and juices in her diet, which provide her all the necessary vitamins, minerals. Her day begins with fruits and eats balanced meals during the day. She has also incorporated intermittent fasting as a lifestyle, which has helped her heal and recover.

She is a role model for all who give up on life after suffering from health issues. She is full of energy, and there is not a single dull moment in her life. I wish her good health and happiness always!

REFERENCES

INTRODUCTION

1. Jahan F, Nanji K, Qidwai W, Qasim R. Fibromyalgia syndrome: an overview of pathophysiology, diagnosis and management. Oman Med J. 2012;27(3):192-195. doi:10.5001/omj.2012.44.

I

1. https://www.iasp-pain.org/PublicationsNews/
2. https://www.practicalpainmanagement.com/pain/myofascial/fda-approves-clinical-trial-fibromyalgia-using-tb-vaccine.
3. Flodin P, Martinsen S, Löfgren M, Bileviciute-Ljungar I, Kosek E, Fransson P. Fibromyalgia is associated with decreased connectivity between pain- and sensorimotor brain areas. Brain Connect. 2014;4(08):587–594.
4. Daniel S. Albrecht, Anton Forsberg, Angelica Sandström, Courtney Bergan, Diana Kadetoff, Ekaterina Protsenko, Jon Lampa, Yvonne C. Lee, Caroline Olgart Höglund, Ciprian Catana, Simon Cervenka, Oluwaseun Akeju, Mats Lekander, George Cohen, Christer Halldin, Norman Taylor, Minhae Kim, Jacob M. Hooker, Robert R. Edwards, Vitaly Napadow, Eva Kosek, Marco L. Loggia. Brain glial activation in fibromyalgia – A multi-site positron emission tomography investigation. Brain, Behavior, and Immunity, 2018; DOI: 10.1016/j.bbi.2018.09.018.
5. Kennel KA, Drake MT, Hurley DL. Vitamin D deficiency in adults: when to test and how to treat. Mayo Clin Proc. 2010;85(8):752-758. doi:10.4065/mcp.2010.0138.

II

1. Suffered Long Enough: A Physician's Journey of Overcoming Fibromyalgia, Chronic Fatigue, and Lyme by MD William C. Rawls Jr and William Rawls.
2. Sephton SE, Salmon P, Weissbecker I, et al. Mindfulness meditation alleviates depressive symptoms in women with fibromyalgia: results of a randomized clinical trial. Arthritis Rheum. 2007;57(1):77-85. doi:10.1002/art.22478.
3. Castro-Sánchez AM, Matarán-Peñarrocha GA, Arroyo-Morales M, Saavedra-Hernández M, Fernández-Sola C, Moreno-Lorenzo C. Effects of myofascial release techniques on pain, physical function, and postural stability in patients with fibromyalgia: a randomized controlled trial. Clin Rehabil. 2011;25(9):800-813. doi:10.1177/0269215511399476.
4. Blunt KL, Rajwani MH, Guerriero RC. The effectiveness of chiropractic management of fibromyalgia patients: a pilot study. J Manipulative Physiol Ther. 1997;20(6):389-399.
5. Adam J. Krause, Aric A. Prather, Tor D. Wager, Martin A. Lindquist, Matthew P. Walker Journal of Neuroscience 20 March 2019, 39 (12) 2291-2300; DOI: 10.1523/JNEUROSCI.2408-18.2018.
6. Andrade, A., de Azevedo Klumb Steffens, R., Sieczkowska, S.M. et al. A systematic review of the effects of strength training in patients with fibromyalgia: clinical outcomes and design considerations. Adv Rheumatol 58, 36 (2018). https://doi.org/10.1186/s42358-018-0033-9

III

1. Miki K, Nakae A, Shi K, et al. Frequency of mental disorders among chronic pain patients with or without fibromyalgia in Japan. Neuropsychopharmacol Rep. 2018;38(4):167-174. doi:10.1002/npr2.12025

IV

1. https://www.sleepfoundation.org/physical-health/pain-and-sleep
2. Study Adam J. Krause, Aric A. Prather, Tor D. Wager, Martin A. Lindquist, Matthew P. Walker Journal of Neuroscience 20 March 2019, 39 (12) 2291-2300; DOI: 10.1523/JNEUROSCI.2408-18.2018

3. Viola-Saltzman M, Watson NF, Bogart A, Goldberg J, Buchwald D. High prevalence of restless legs syndrome among patients with fibromyalgia: a controlled cross-sectional study. J Clin Sleep Med. 2010;6(5):423-427.
4. https://www.mayoclinic.org/diseases-conditions/insomnia/in-depth/insomnia-treatment/art-20046677

V

1. Triadafilopoulos G, Simms RW, Goldenberg DL. Bowel dysfunction in fibromyalgia syndrome. Dig Dis Sci 1991;36:59–64.
2. Wallace DJ, Hallegua DS. Fibromyalgia: the gastrointestinal link. Curr Pain Headache Rep. 2004 Oct;8(5):364-8. doi: 10.1007/s11916-996-0009-z. PMID: 15361320.
3. https://www.healthline.com/health/fibromyalgia-and-ibs#fibromyalgia-and-ibs-connection
4. Chang L. The association of functional gastrointestinal disorders and fibromyalgia. Eur J Surg Suppl. 1998;(583):32-6. doi: 10.1080/11024159850191210. PMID: 10027670.
5. Erdrich, Sharon & Hawrelak, Jason & Myers, Stephen & Harnett, Joanna. Determining the association between fibromyalgia, the gut microbiome and its biomarkers: A systematic review. BMC Muscul Dis 2020. 21. 10.1186/s12891-020-03201-9.
6. Pimentel M, Wallace D, Hallegua D, Chow E, Kong Y, Park S, Lin HC. A link between irritable bowel syndrome and fibromyalgia may be related to findings on lactulose breath testing. Ann Rheum Dis. 2004 Apr;63(4):450-2. doi: 10.1136/ard.2003.011502. PMID: 15020342; PMCID: PMC1754959.
7. Slim, M., Calandre, E.P. & Rico-Villademoros, F. An insight into the gastrointestinal component of fibromyalgia: clinical manifestations and potential underlying mechanisms. Rheumatol Int 35, 433–444 (2015). https://doi.org/10.1007/s00296-014-3109-9
8. Wallace DJ, Hallegua DS. Fibromyalgia: the gastrointestinal link. Curr Pain Headache Rep. 2004 Oct;8(5):364-8. doi: 10.1007/s11916-996-0009-z. PMID: 15361320.
9. Triadafilopoulos G, Simms RW, Goldenberg DL. Bowel dysfunction in fibromyalgia syndrome. Dig Dis Sci 1991;36:59–64

VI

1. J.N. Ablin, D. Buskila. Predicting fibromyalgia, a narrative review: Are we better thanfools and children? Eur J Pain 18 2014; 1060–1066.
2. Arout CA, Sofuoglu M, Bastian LA, Rosenheck RA. Gender Differences in the Prevalence of Fibromyalgia and in Concomitant Medical and Psychiatric Disorders: A National Veterans Health Administration Study. J Womens Health (Larchmt). 2018;27(8):1035-1044. doi:10.1089/jwh.2017.6622
3. Bäckryd E, Tanum L, Lind AL, Larsson A, Gordh T. Evidence of both systemic inflammation and neuroinflammation in fibromyalgia patients, as assessed by a multiplex protein panel applied to the cerebrospinal fluid and to plasma. J Pain Res. 2017;10:515-525. Published 2017 Mar 3. doi:10.2147/JPR.S128508
4. J.N. Ablin, D. Buskila. Predicting fibromyalgia, a narrative review: Are we better thanfools and children? Eur J Pain 18 2014; 1060–1066.
5. Mork PJ, Nilsen TI. Sleep problems and risk of fibromyalgia: longitudinal data on an adult female population in Norway. Arthritis Rheum. 2012 Jan;64(1):281-4. doi: 10.1002/art.33346. PMID: 22081440.
6. http://www.anaturalhealingcenter.com/documents/Thorne/articles/InfluenzaAndFibromyalgia.pdf
7. Krumina A, Chapenko S, Kenina V, et al. The role of HHV-6 and HHV-7 infections in the development of fibromyalgia [published correction appears in J Neurovirol. 2019 Jan 24;:]. J Neurovirol. 2019;25(2):194-207. doi:10.1007/s13365-018-0703-8
8. Taylor AG, Adelstein KE, Fischer-White TG, Murugesan M, Anderson JG. Perspectives on Living With Fibromyalgia. Glob Qual Nurs Res. 2016;3:2333393616658141. Published 2016 Jul 6. doi:10.1177/2333393616658141
9. Ablin JN, Buskila D. Predicting fibromyalgia, a narrative review: are we better than fools and children? Eur J Pain. 2014 Sep;18(8):1060-6. doi: 10.1002/j.1532-2149.2014.00481.x. Epub 2014 Mar 11. PMID: 24619570.
10. Mork PJ, Nilsen TI. Sleep problems and risk of fibromyalgia: longitudinal data on an adult female population in Norway. Arthritis Rheum. 2012 Jan;64(1):281-4. doi: 10.1002/art.33346. PMID: 22081440.

VII

1. https://files.nccih.nih.gov/s3fs-public/Fibromyalgia_11-08-2015.pdf
2. Guzzo M, Iannuccelli C, Gerardi M, et alAB0925 Gender difference in fibromyalgia: comparison between male and female patients from an italian monocentric cohortAnnals of the Rheumatic Diseases 2017;76:1379
3. Yunus, M.B. The role of gender in fibromyalgia syndrome. Curr Rheumatol Rep 3, 128–134 (2001). https://doi.org/10.1007/s11926-001-0008-3

VIII

1. Okifuji A, Turk DC. Sex hormones and pain in regularly menstruating women with fibromyalgia syndrome. J Pain.
2. White HD, Brown LA, Gyurik RJ, et al. Treatment of pain in fibromyalgia patients with testosterone gel: Pharmacokinetics and clinical response. Int Immunopharmacol. 2015;27(2):249-256. doi:10.1016/j.intimp.2015.05.016
3. Kashikar-Zuck S, Ting TV. Juvenile fibromyalgia: current status of research and future developments. Nat Rev Rheumatol. 2014;10(2):89-96. doi:10.1038/nrrheum.2013.177
4. Genç H, Atasever M, Duyur Çakit B, Seval M, Koç A. The Effects of Fibromyalgia Syndrome on Physical Function and Psychological Status of Pregnant Females. Arch Rheumatol. 2017;32(2):129-140. Published 2017 Jan 5. doi:10.5606/ArchRheumatol.2017.6028

X

1. https://www.practicalpainmanagement.com/patient/conditions/fibromyalgia/physical-therapy-fibromyalgia#:~:text=By%20using%20safe%2C%20gentle%2C%20and,treatments%2C%20such%20as%20flexibility%20exercises
2. Li YH, Wang FY, Feng CQ, Yang XF, Sun YH. Massage therapy for fibromyalgia: a systematic review and meta-analysis of randomised controlled trials. PLoS One. 2014;9(2):e89304. Published 2014 Feb 20. doi:10.1371/journal.pone.0089304
3. Yuan SL, Berssaneti AA, Marques AP. Effects of shiatsu in the management of fibromyalgia symptoms: a controlled pilot

study. J Manipulative PhysiolTher. 2013;36(7):436-443. doi:10.1016/j.jmpt.2013.05.019

4. Verma A, Shete SU, Doddoli G. Yoga therapy for fibromyalgia syndrome: A case report. J Family Med Prim Care. 2020;9(1):435-438. Published 2020 Jan 28. doi:10.4103/jfmpc.jfmpc_816_19
5. https://www.sciencedaily.com/releases/2010/10/101014083119.htm

XI

1. Donaldson MS, Speight N, Loomis S. Fibromyalgia syndrome improved using a mostly raw vegetarian diet: an observational study. BMC Complement Altern Med. 2001;1:7. doi:10.1186/1472-6882-1-7
2. Kaartinen K, Lammi K, Hypen M, Nenonen M, Hanninen O, Rauma AL. Vegan diet alleviates fibromyalgia symptoms. Scand J Rheumatol. 2000;29(5):308-13. doi: 10.1080/030097400447697. PMID: 11093597.
3. https://asitis.com/17/8-10.html

XII

1. Wolfe F, Smythe HA, Yunus MB, Bennett RM, Bombardier C, Goldenberg DL, Tugwell P, Campbell SM, Abeles M, Clark P, et al. The American College of Rheumatology 1990 Criteria for the Classification of Fibromyalgia. Report of the Multicenter Criteria Committee. Arthritis Rheum. 1990 Feb;33(2):160-72. doi: 10.1002/art.1780330203. PMID: 2306288.
2. Wolfe F, Clauw DJ, Fitzcharles MA, Goldenberg DL, Katz RS, Mease P, Russell AS, Russell IJ, Winfield JB, Yunus MB. The American College of Rheumatology preliminary diagnostic criteria for fibromyalgia and measurement of symptom severity. Arthritis Care Res (Hoboken). 2010 May;62(5):600-10. doi: 10.1002/acr.20140. PMID: 20461783.

Printed in the USA
CPSIA information can be obtained
at www.ICGtesting.com
LVHW091435251123
764907LV00006B/344